professions

CHURCHILL LIVINGSTONE NURSING TEXTS

Nutrition and Dietetics for Nurses
Fifth edition
Mary E. Beck

Practical Notes on Nursing Procedures
Seventh edition
J. D. Britten

Bacteriology and Immunity for Nurses
Fifth edition
Ronald Hare and E. Mary Cooke

Drugs and Pharmacology for Nurses
Seventh edition
S. J. Hopkins

Essentials of Paediatrics for Nurses
Fifth edition
I. Kessel

Psychology as Applied to Nursing
Seventh edition
Andrew McGhie

A Nurse's Guide to Anaesthetics, Resuscitation and Intensive Care
Sixth edition
Walter Norris and D. Campbell

Anatomy and Physiology Applied to Nursing
Fifth edition
Janet T. E. Riddle

Principles of Nursing
Second edition
Nancy Roper

Foundations of Nursing and First Aid
Fifth edition
Janet S. Ross and Kathleen J. W. Wilson

Sociology and Nursing
First edition
James P. Smith

Pharmacology for Nurses
Seventh edition
J. R. Trounce

Practical Therapeutics for Nursing and related professions

James A. Boyle
MD(Glas.) MRCP(Ed. and Lond.)
Formerly Lecturer in Medicine,
Royal Infirmary, Glasgow

Revised by

David A. Henry MB ChB MRCP
Lecturer, Department of Therapeutics
University of Nottingham, Nottingham

William R. Greig MB ChB FRCP(Ed.) FRCP(Glas.)
Formerly Consultant Physician,
Department of Nuclear Medicine,
Royal Infirmary, Glasgow

THIRD EDITION

CHURCHILL LIVINGSTONE
EDINBURGH LONDON AND NEW YORK 1900

CHURCHILL LIVINGSTONE
Medical Division of the Longman Group Limited

Distributed in the United States of America by Churchill Livingstone Inc., 19 West 44th Street, New York, N.Y. 10036, and by associated companies, branches and representatives throughout the world.

First edition 1967
Second edition 1974
Third edition 1980

First and 2nd edition published under title:
Lecture Notes in Pharmacology and Therapeutics for Nurses

ISBN 0 443 01540 6

British Library Cataloguing in Publication Data
Boyle, James Anthony
 Practical therapeutics for nursing and
 related professions. — 3rd ed. — (Churchill
 Livingstcre nursing texts).
 1. Pharmacology
 I. Title   II. Henry, David A   III. Greig,
 William Rattray   IV. Lecture notes in
 pharmacology and therapeutics for
 nurses
 615'.7'024613   RM125   80-40097

Printed in Singapore
by Singapore Offset Printing Pte Ltd

Preface to the Third Edition

This third edition of Dr. James Boyle's book, formerly known as *Lecture Notes in Pharmacology and Therapeutics for Nurses*, has been completely reorganised and rewritten, and a 'disease-orientated' approach has been adopted. This reorganisation was thought to be desirable for many reasons. Changes have occurred in the types of drugs now available and also in the manner in which some of the older remedies are used. Furthermore, it is a characteristic of modern therapy that individual drugs may be used successfully to treat several quite different conditions, and both the method of administration and dosage may change. An example is adrenergic blocking drugs which are prescribed in angina, hypertension, cardiac arrhythmias and for the symptomatic treatment of thyrotoxicosis.

As a result of this new approach, and as befits a textbook of therapeutics, drugs of different types appear grouped together under the indication of their use (e.g. cardiac failure or anaemia) rather than by strict pharmacological classification. Inevitably, certain agents are covered several times in different sections of the book. The basic mode of action is, however, usually discussed only once, and the index and cross references in the text should guide the reader.

The new approach taken for this edition inevitably meant that the titles and content of each chapter had to be re-thought and re-ordered. The amount of alteration, rearrangement and addition of new material varied from one chapter to the other, although nearly all have been extensively revised. Completely new chapters include those on pain (7) malignant disease (10) and intravenous fluid therapy (12). The section on mode of action of drugs in Chapter 1 has been expanded, as has the section devoted to adverse drug effects in Chapter 13. Where therapy is complex and sometimes controversial a brief outline of broad therapeutic approach is provided under 'principles of management of . . .'.

It is hoped that this book will give to the reader a useful outline of modern therapeutic practice. Of course it in no way constitutes an exhaustive list of all available drugs and doses. When the reader is in doubt he or she should consult the British National Formulary (B.N.F.), the Monthly Index of Medical Specialties (M.I.M.S.) or standard pharmacological texts.

Nottingham, 1980   D.A.H

Preface to the First Edition

Pharmacology (the study of the mode of action of drugs) and therapeutics (the art of using drugs to cure disease or alleviate suffering) are two of the most exciting branches of internal medicine. Too often, however, both of these gripping disciplines lose any interest they may initially have held for the nurse as she grapples with a long list of dosages and side effects. I believe that the study of pharmacology and therapeutics is not a matter of learning doses of drugs: the nurse is not called upon to prescribe in Great Britain and for this reason a knowledge of the dose of a drug is unnecessary; in any case constant use will familiarize her with the correct doses of the commonly prescribed drugs. Side effects on the other hand will often be recognized first by the nurse as she sees much more of her patient than any doctor. For this reason I have tried to describe side effects not as lists to be remembered but rather as events which happen to patients, events which in themselves may be serious or trivial—but are always interesting.

The book, which is based on lectures delivered at Glasgow Royal Infirmary, is not intended as a reference manual. My aim has been to highlight the *principles* underlying the administration of the more commonly used drugs.

I am grateful to my long suffering wife for her encouragement and especially for her forbearance while this book was in preparation.

1967   James A. Boyle

Contents

Note

Our knowledge in clinical medicine and related biological sciences is constantly changing. As new information obtained from clinical experience and research becomes available, changes in treatment and in the use of drugs become necessary. The authors and the publisher of this volume have, as far as it is possible to do so, taken care to make certain that the doses of drugs and schedules of treatment are accurate and compatible with the standards generally accepted at the time of publication. The readers are advised, however, to consult carefully. the instruction and information material included in the package insert of each drug or therapeutic agent that they plan to administer in order to make certain that there have been no changes in the recommended dose of the drug or the indications or contraindications for its administration. This precaution is especially important when using new or infrequently used drugs.

Mode of action of drugs and methods of administration

INTRODUCTION

Since earliest times man has endeavoured to find remedies for the many diseases which afflict the human body. The majority of early remedies were extracts of herbs and plants and their discovery was a process of trial and error. Most were probably ineffective but a few, for instance poppy seeds (opium) and foxglove (digitalis), produced a dramatic response, and derivatives of these are still widely used today. Although we have known for centuries that these drugs are effective, their precise mode of action has remained something of a mystery. It is only in the last few years that the science of pharmacology has provided us with some of the answers.

MODE OF ACTION OF DRUGS—RECEPTOR THEORY

Most modern drugs, and indeed many of the older remedies, are complex chemical compounds. To have an effect they must enter the body where they are carried to their site of action in the blood stream. In the blood most drugs are carried partly attached to the plasma proteins, usually albumin, and partly dissolved in the water content of the plasma (in solution). Usually it is the unbound fraction which is active and drug molecules in solution probably combine with special receptors on the surface of the body cells (Fig 1.1). This combination of drug and receptor may then trigger a response. Sometimes the drug molecule itself is not active, but by occupying a receptor site may block the attachment of a naturally occurring active substance (Fig. 1.2). Examples of this are atropine blocking the effect of acetylcholine on the gut or propranolol blocking the effect of adrenaline on the heart. This is known as 'competitive antagonism' and is the basis of action of many effective drugs. A modern example is the new anti-ulcer remedy cimetidine which binds to receptors in the stomach and so blocks the attachment of histamine molecules, thereby reducing the secretion of acid. The official name for this drug therefore is an H^2 (histamine) receptor antagonist. Sometimes drugs must enter the cell to have an effect. Corticosteroids are thought to combine with steroid receptor sites within the cell and produce a response by altering the rate of synthesis of special proteins. By doing this they can have a fundamental effect on inflammation in certain tissues.

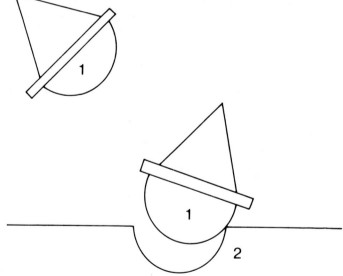

Fig. 1.1 Simplified representation of drug molecules (1) interacting with a tissue receptor (2). In this case the 'drug' is the naturally occurring compound histamine. There are two types of histamine receptor in the body. This is an H^2 receptor in the stomach and the action of histamine here is to increase gastric acid secretion.

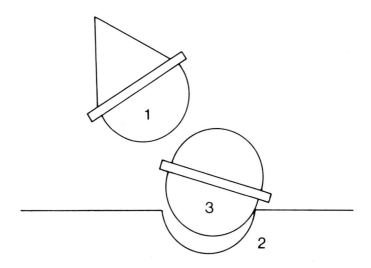

Fig. 1.2 In this case a therapeutic compound (3)—the H^2 receptor antagonist drug cimetidine—is binding to an H^2 receptor in the stomach, thus 'blocking' the action of histamine. Note that the drug has a similar but not identical structure to that of histamine. By blocking the action of histamine cimetidine reduces gastric acid secretion and aids healing of peptic ulcers (see Chapter 2). With acknowledgements to Smith Kline & French Ltd.

Almost all drugs act in a reversible fashion. That is, when we stop giving the drug to the patient its concentration in the body falls, the drug receptors become unoccupied and the therapeutic effect wears off.

When giving a drug to a patient we are usually looking for a sustained response. For instance a drug given for the treatment of epilepsy would be of no value if it only worked for say 8 hours in the day. Our aim in such cases is to ensure that a sufficient number of tissue receptors are in contact with the correct concentration of the drug throughout the day. It must be said that there are exceptions to this rule: some antibacterial and anticancer drugs are thought to act most effectively in a 'hit and run' fashion. By this we mean that they have an intense action, producing death of bacteria or malignant cells over a short period before the drug is eliminated from the body (these drugs are usually eliminated quickly). The reasons for this mode of action are not fully understood but in the case of anticancer remedies, high concentrations of drug over a long period will damage normal tissue as well as the cancer cells.

This account of the mode of drug action is certainly an oversimplification. The exact means by which many drugs produce their effect and the best methods of using them have not yet been determined. Much work remains to be done in this area.

BODY HANDLING OF DRUGS

Before using drugs in an intelligent fashion we must know how the body eliminates them. Some substances for instance frusemide, digoxin and many antibacterial agents are excreted by the kidney virtually unchanged. Others, for instance diazepam, phenytoin and phenylbutazone, undergo extensive alteration of their chemical structure in the liver prior to excretion from the body. This process is known as drug metabolism. In most cases the drug metabolites have no therapeutic action, so we say that these drugs are inactivated in the liver. This knowledge is important because in general individuals with normal kidneys will not vary a great deal in the speed with which they excrete an unchanged drug (e.g. digoxin). If the kidneys are known to be damaged then the renal function can be estimated by various tests and an appropriate change made to the dosage of the drug to prevent excessive accumulation and toxicity. With drugs that are inactivated by the liver, however, the situation is very different. Individuals with healthy livers vary greatly in the speed with which they metabolise certain drugs and there are no tests available which allow us to differentiate easily between those who inactivate the drug quickly and those who do so slowly. This means that a fixed dose of a drug, say 100 mg of the antiepileptic drug phenytoin every 8 hours may be too much for one patient and result in side effects whereas another patient who inactivates the drug quickly will not retain enough in the body to have a proper effect and will continue to have seizures.

The situation is made even more complicated by the fact that drugs themselves vary greatly in the speed with which they are eliminated from the body. For instance procainamide (used in cardiac arrhythmias) is excreted partly by the liver and partly by the kidneys in a matter of a few hours, while phenytoin may take days to disappear from the body. In practice this means that in order to keep the concentration of procainamide in the blood stream, and therefore in the heart, at the right level, the drug must be given to the patient frequently—say six times a day. By contrast phenytoin can be administered as seldom as once a day and still have an effect.

This makes the whole business of giving a drug to a patient sound very complicated. Fortunately for a large number of drugs in common use it does not seem essential to provide the body with a precise quantity in order to be effective, so that our normal rather thoughtless habit of providing exactly the same dose for every patient still produces results. There is, however, a growing list of drugs, including digoxin, procainamide, phenytoin, lithium and gentamicin which seem to require a fairly precise concentration in the body to have their effect. When using these drugs therefore it is necessary to 'tailor' the dose for each individual patient and measurement of the concentration of drug in the blood stream is helpful in ensuring a good therapeutic response while avoiding serious toxicity.

It should always be borne in mind that when a patient fails to respond to treatment it may not be the fault of the drug but failure on behalf of the medical attendants to ensure that the right amount of drug has reached the right tissues at the right time.

METHODS OF ADMINISTRATION

Before discussing the ways in which drugs are administered to patients, a few general comments on your attitude to the patients whom you are treating are necessary. Patients are apprehensive of the sights, sounds and smells of a hospital. Many of them are frightened of injections or of unfamiliar medicines and some of them have their response to a drug affected by the nurse's attitude to them and to their treatment. It is not unknown for a hypnotic tablet to fail to produce sleep because of the patient's anxieties about the tablet and the effect it will have on him, or because of the unsympathetic manner in which it was given to him. The power of suggestion is very strong, especially where the ill patient is concerned. A skilful nurse has been known to induce sleep in a patient by the administration of paracetamol tablets and the confident suggestion that these will help him get off to sleep. From these two examples it is clear that your attitude to your patient and his treatment is of the greatest importance irrespective of the drug you are giving him. One word of explanation from you before you give your patient a tablet or injection is of great value in allaying his fears and speeding his recovery or response to treatment.

Oral administration of drugs

Orally administered substances may be absorbed into the blood stream through the oral mucous membrane (buccal mucosa), through the stomach or through the small bowel. They then circulate in the blood stream and are carried to the part of the body they are to act upon.

Absorption through the buccal mucosa

It is important that you know that two commonly used drugs are absorbed in this manner; glyceryl trinitrate, used in the treatment of angina pectoris and testosterone which is used in male androgen deficiency. If these drugs are swallowed they are rapidly broken down to inert substances in the stomach. It follows that if your patient does swallow them he will obtain no benefit from his treatment. Accordingly, you should ensure that he is aware that these drugs have to be placed underneath the tongue and kept there while they dissolve. An alternative method of giving testosterone is by regular monthly injection.

Absorption through the stomach

Surprisingly, few drugs are absorbed to any great extent from the stomach, as the type of mucosa and the extreme acidity create unsuitable conditions.

·One substance which is partly absorbed from the stomach is alcohol which may be detected in the blood stream as little as 5 minutes after ingestion. The absorption of alcohol in this way is slowed down if there is food in the stomach, especially fat containing foods. The corollary of this statement is that alcohol is absorbed extremely rapidly and in appreciable quantities on an empty stomach. Aspirin and phenylbutazone also undergo some absorption in the stomach and this is because they are themselves acidic compounds and the environment is suitable.

Absorption from the small intestine

The great majority of drugs are absorbed into the blood steam from the small intestine. Absorption of most drugs is not an active process but occurs by simple diffusion of the chemical across the cell membrane of the intestinal mucosa. There are many factors which influence the rate of absorption and the amount of drug absorbed from the small bowel.

Many substances cannot be absorbed at all because they are inactivated by enzymes in the small bowel. A good example of this is insulin, which is rapidly broken down in the bowel to inert fragments and is therefore inactive when given orally. Another example of a substance which cannot be absorbed on its own orally is the drug hydroxycobalamin or vitamin B12 which is given to treat patients who suffer from pernicious anaemia. In health the stomach produces a substance called intrinsic factor which couples up with the small amounts of vitamin B12 obtained in the diet. The intrinsic factor allows vitamin B12 to be absorbed in the distal ileum and from there it is taken in the blood stream to the bone marrow where it is essential for the production of red blood cells. In pernicious anaemia, however, the stomach fails to secrete intrinsic factor and the vitamin B12 which is in the diet then fails to be absorbed. Even when the vitamin is given in massive doses by mouth to patients with pernicious anaemia they fail to absorb it, and it is therefore necessary to give it by injection.

Even under normal conditions individuals vary greatly in their ability to absorb drugs from the small intestine. There are many reasons for this, but differences in gastrointestinal motility and the presence of foodstuffs or other drugs are particularly important. It should be remembered that following absorption drugs enter the portal vein and must pass through the liver to reach other parts of the body. The liver is capable of 'mopping up' large quantities of certain drugs e.g. propranolol. This is termed 'first pass clearance' and it may greatly reduce the amount of drug which finally reaches its target organ. During ill health any factor which causes slow emptying of the stomach contents into the small bowel will cause drugs to be absorbed slowly. Patients who are severely ill or who are shocked from loss of blood or severe pain (as in myocardial infarction or gallstone colic) may exhibit slow gastric emptying. For this reason shocked patients are not usually given drugs orally. Febrile conditions, too, are known to decrease the absorption of drugs and this is especially so in children. From this you can see that the oral absorption of drugs may be slowed or erratic or uncertain. If it is desired that a drug produce a rapid action in a patient who is very ill, a strong case can be made out in many instances for giving that drug by injection. If a sustained action is required, however, in a patient who is less ill and especially if treatment is to be prolonged, then differences in absorption may be permissible and the drug can be given orally.

The advantages of oral administration are fairly obvious. Swallowing a tablet is always preferable to receiving an injection, particularly if the drug has to be administered regularly and treatment has to be continued over a long period. Oral administration is really the only satisfactory solution for patients continuing treatment at home. Finally, side effects tend to be less severe as the concentration of drug in the body following absorption from the intestine is lower than that following parenteral administration.

Parenteral administration of drugs

When a drug is administered other than locally or by the alimentary tract it is said to be given *parenterally*. In practice this usually means that the drug is given by subcutaneous, intramuscular or intravenous injection (intrathecal injection of a substance into the cerebrospinal fluid in the subarachnoid space is also covered by the term). Parenteral administration has three advantages over the alimentary route:

1. There is increased certainty of absorption. The certainty of absorption varies with whether the drug is given subcutaneously, intramuscularly or intravenously as is discussed below
2. Absorption of the drug is more rapid than with oral administration
3. The possibility of destruction of the drug in the bowel or in the liver (first pass clearance) is avoided by parenteral administration.

Subcutaneous injection

This is a procedure which is relatively simple and which can therefore be taught to patients so that they may perform injections upon themselves. Almost all diabetic patients requiring insulin treatment, for example, are taught to inject their insulin subcutaneously once or twice a day. There is little danger of vital structures such as nerves or arteries being pierced when a subcutaneous injection is given but you must remind your patient to draw back the plunger of the syringe after he has inserted the needle under the skin prior to injecting the contents. This manoeuvre lets him see whether or not he has inadvertently placed the point of the needle in a small superficial vein and will safeguard him from injecting his drug intravenously. Inadvertent intravenous injection of a local anaesthetic such as xylocaine or a substance such as adrenalin can happen all too easily in the belief that it is a subcutaneous injection and this can have disastrous results. What you teach your diabetic patients to do, you should therefore practise yourself. When giving a subcutaneous injection *always* check that the tip of the needle is not in a vein. If it is in the vein you will see this when a little blood enters the syringe on withdrawing the plunger slightly.

When a drug is deposited in the subcutaneous tissues it normally diffuses quite rapidly into the adjacent venules and arterioles and it is thus carried throughout the body in the blood stream. In shocked patients, however, the venules and arterioles in the subcutaneous tissues become constricted and a drug injected subcutaneously may diffuse extremely slowly or not at all into these constricted blood vessels. Under these conditions large pools of drug lie in the subcutaneous tissue and are of little benefit to the patient.

For example, a patient in severe diabetic coma, given all of his insulin by subcutaneous injection may show no fall in his blood sugar because of failure of the insulin to be absorbed. There is, in addition, the danger that when this patient does recover (for example, after insulin has been given intravenously at a later date), the insulin lying subcutaneously may be then absorbed into the blood stream and cause hypoglycaemia.

For these reasons it is wiser to avoid subcutaneous injections in shocked or severely ill patients in whom peripheral vasoconstriction may be expected. In these patients the deep intramuscular or intravenous route should be chosen for parenteral administration.

Intramuscular injection

This is a very useful route of drug administration.

Many of the muscles of the human body are traversed by nerves, arteries and large veins. You will find that patients are curiously ungrateful to have these structures injected. If you give a patient an intramuscular injection of penicillin to cure a boil and you unwittingly inject the drug into the sciatic nerve thus giving him foot drop (to mention nothing of the pain) he will not thank you. There are three muscle sites which can be injected without fear of an accident of this sort happening. They are:

1. The upper and outer quadrant of the buttock
2. The outer side of the thigh, two or three inches below the greater trochanter (approximately 5 to 7 cm)
3. The mid-deltoid region.

These sites are illustrated diagrammatically in Figure 1.3. Many nurses tend to inject further and further anteriorly when they are injecting into the thigh. This practice is to be avoided at all costs as there is a grave danger of hitting the femoral artery which runs down the anterior aspect of the thigh.

The description of the technique of good intramuscular injection is beyond the scope of this book and in any case it is not a technique which is learned by reading about it but by constant practice in the wards.

The same precautions must be observed for intramuscular injection as for subcutaneous injection. *Always* check that the tip of your needle is not lying in a small vein before injecting.

Water soluble drugs such as benzyl penicillin are absorbed quite rapidly after deep intramuscular injection and adequate blood levels of drug can be attained 1 to 3 hours later. There are many other substances which are prepared as non-water soluble compounds or as suspensions which are similarly slowly absorbed following intramuscular injection and therefore have a long duration of action, e.g. insulin zinc suspension.

Intravenous injection

In Great Britain you will not normally be called upon to administer drugs by intravenous injection. In some special units trained nurses are called upon to give drugs by this route and you should therefore be familiar with the advantages of this technique. In most medical wards a vein in the antecubital fossa or forearm is chosen for intravenous injection. The anaesthetist, however, finds it more convenient to use the veins on the dorsum of the hand. He can thus inject drugs intravenously during the operation without getting in the way of the surgeon or his assistants.

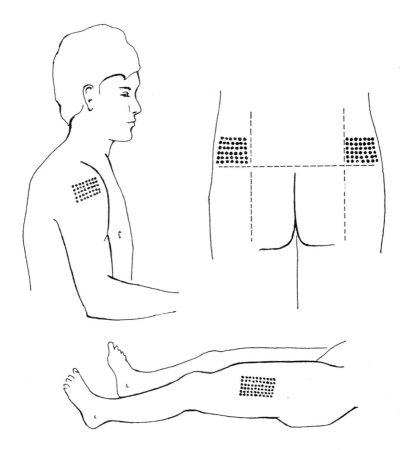

Fig. 1.3. Sites for intramuscular injection: mid-deltoid, buttock and thigh region (stippled areas).

Intravenous injections have the advantage of producing a very rapid effect because the injected drug mingles instantly with the blood stream. There is thus absolute certainty of absorption. In addition, extremely irritant drugs which might cause gastric intolerance when given orally, or muscle necrosis when given intramuscularly, can be safely administered intravenously. You might at first think this statement rather odd. The explanation is that irritant substances are quickly diluted in the fast flowing blood stream and when they are slowly injected intravenously their irritant properties are vastly reduced. Mustine, a drug used in the treatment of malignant disease, is so irritant that it can cause blistering of the intact skin. It is administered intravenously to ensure its rapid dilution in the blood stream and is usually given slowly into the tubing of an intravenous infusion set which is delivering fluid at a fast rate into a vein.

There are some disadvantages in intravenous injection. The drug may be rapidly utilised in the blood stream necessitating frequent injections at short intervals. This is well illustrated by patients with diabetic coma who are treated with intravenous insulin. These patients may require injections of insulin at hourly intervals. This has resulted in techniques by which insulin is administered by continuous infusion either injected into the bottles of fluid or delivered by an electrically driven pump. Local thombosis of the vein may be produced by careless or inexperienced operators or by the too rapid injection of irritant solutions. Should the injected solution extravasate outside the vein, necrosis of the tissues can occur. Finally, if the wrong drug or too much of the correct drug is administered, one has very little time to take corrective measures or administer an antidote before damage is done.

Intrathecal injection

This route is used when a high concentration of drug is desired within the cerebrospinal fluid or within the brain in as short a time as possible. Many drugs diffuse poorly and slowly from the blood stream into the cerebrospinal fluid. It is as if there were an invisible barrier which hinders diffusion from the blood stream into this fluid and thence into the brain. Indeed the phenomenon of poor diffusion from blood to brain tissue is said to be caused by the 'blood-brain barrier' although it is not possible to show the anatomical existence of such a barrier. In order to achieve therapeutic concentrations of drug in the cerebrospinal fluid, one must either achieve astronomically high levels of drug in the blood stream or give the drug by intrathecal injection. Patients with tuberculous meningitis are often initially treated by intrathecal injections of streptomycin.

One class of drug which diffuses very readily into the cerebrospinal fluid is the sulphonamides and because of this these agents are still used in the treatment of meningococcal meningitis. Sulphonamides must *never* be given intrathecally because they cause an intense inflammatory reaction round the spinal cord which leads to spinal cord damage and paralysis.

Administration of drugs by inhalation

Some drugs are administered in the form of gases or tiny droplets of solution which are inhaled by the patient. Gases such as halothane or nitrous oxide are administered usually by anaesthetists. In Great Britain the nurse is not called upon to administer anaesthetic gases. Once the gas has been inhaled it passes to the alveoli of the lung whence it is absorbed into the lung capillaries. From there the gas gains access to the cerebral blood stream where it exerts its effect.

Other than in anaesthetics the administration of drugs by inhalation is confined to the treatment of asthma. Drugs used in the treatment of bronchospasm, e.g. isoprenaline, salbutamol and more recently corticosteroids can be given by this route. The patient inhales the fine mist of the drug (a mixture of tiny droplets of solution and air) which is dispensed from a special aerosol. The drug then passes to the bronchi and bronchioles where it exerts a local effect by producing dilatation of these structures.

Absorption through the rectum

The practice of administering drugs by suppository or enema is more widespread on the continent of Europe than in Great Britain. In the United Kingdom a few drugs, aminophylline and indomethicin being the best examples, are given by this route on the basis that absorption into the body is slower, producing a more sustained effect, and side effects such as gastric irritation and ulceration are less. There may be some truth in these statements but research has revealed that this is a very unreliable means of giving drugs as absorption is very poor from this site. Patients are often intolerant of suppositories and side effects such as local irritation of the rectum may occur. Rectal administration of drugs is in general not recommended.

Local administration of drugs

Local administration of a drug means that the drug is brought into immediate contact with the area to be treated. In practice this method is used most frequently in treatment of skin conditions and an account of the variety and types of drugs used in dermatology is outside the scope of this book. The most effective drugs which act locally on skin are corticosteroids, and in the past decade there has been a marked increase in the use of such drugs. Although often dramatically effective, potent steroids used over a long period may damage the skin, may encourage fungal infections and may even be absorbed through inflamed skin in sufficient quantities to produce side effects on other parts of the body. As well as skin, mucus membranes may be accessible to local treatment. Local anaesthetics such as benzocaine can be administered by lozenge or spray to reduce sensation prior to some operative procedure. Antifungal drugs such as nystatin and amphotericin will eradicate monilial infections of the throat or vagina without being absorbed into the body. In this respect it should be noted that antibiotic and antiseptic agents are not nearly so successful in treating bacterial infections either of mucus membranes or skin.

Finally, the inflamed rectum and colonic mucosa of ulcerative colitis can be treated successfully by steroid enemeta and this will reduce the severe side effects associated with giving large doses of these drugs orally or parenterally.

2

Drugs used in the treatment of gastrointestinal diseases

Many drugs administered for gastrointestinal disorders act locally within the lumen of the bowel but a number require to be absorbed and passed through the circulation into the vessels supplying the stomach or intestine before they can be effective.

ANTACIDS

These are amongst the most widely used drugs in the community being available both on prescription and across the counter. They are specifically indicated for the symptomatic treatment of peptic ulcer, but tend also to be used for non-specific and sometimes self-induced disturbances of gastrointestinal function. The pain of peptic ulcer appears to be exacerbated by hydrochloric acid and antacid drugs produce reliable if sometimes short-lived relief of symptoms in most sufferers from this common condition. Their exact mode of action is not clear but they probably act partly by neutralising the acid and partly by acting as a physical barrier between the acid and the ulcer. In the quantities normally taken by ulcer patients antacids merely relieve symptoms but there is some evidence that large doses, particularly if combined with bed rest and cessation of smoking, may reduce secretion of acid and promote healing. The pain of peptic ulcer is periodic with long spells of freedom and most patients only use antacids during painful periods. It is often forgotten that the presence of food within the stomach also produces relief of pain and patients with peptic ulcer should therefore be encouraged to take their antacids when the stomach is empty, in other words between meals. You will often hear them advised to take the drugs after food, and this is unlikely to be of any benefit. There are many of these substances available. The following are the most effective and therefore the most widely used:

1. Sodium bicarbonate
2. Magnesium trisilicate
3. Aluminium hydroxide
4. Milk.

Sodium bicarbonate

This is the quickest-acting antacid which is known. It acts within seconds by neutralising hydrochloric acid to sodium chloride, carbon dioxide and water. The carbon dioxide is sometimes brought up as a tremendous belch by less socially conscious patients.

Sodium bicarbonate is in many ways a very satisfactory antacid but it has two disadvantages. It has a transient action and its prolonged use in overdosage can lead to alkalosis. This is hardly surprising when you remember that this drug is itself an alkali. It is by virtue of this fact that it neutralises hydrochloric acid so rapidly and so effectively. The dose is 1 to 4 g. On account of these disadvantages patients should be encouraged to keep sodium bicarbonate as a standby for the emergency treatment of acute pain and to use another antacid for routine use. Because of the risks of overuse of this drug it is seldom prescribed nowadays for peptic ulcer.

Magnesium trisilicate

This is an insoluble powder. It forms the main ingredient of many proprietary powders. It adsorbs hydrochloric acid in the stomach and in this process it is eventually converted to magnesium carbonate which has a mild purgative effect. Many patients who take magnesium trisilicate thus experience mild diarrhoea. The dose of this drug is 0.5 to 2 g. It has a much longer action than sodium bicarbonate.

Aluminium hydroxide

This is available in tablet form or can be given as a liquid. It reacts with hydrochloric acid and after a series of other reactions in the bowel is converted to aluminium phosphate which has a mild constipating effect. It is a very good antacid especially for treating patients with acute exacerbation of ulcer.

Sometimes magnesium trisilicate is combined with aluminium hydroxide in the hope that the purgative effect of the one will cancel the constipating effect of the other.

Milk

This seemingly simple substance is an extremely efficient antacid by reason of its action as a buffer. A buffer is a substance which can absorb acid or alkali without undergoing changes in its own acidity or alkalinity. Although they may not know why milk is effective in relieving their ulcer pain, many patients have made the empirical discovery that it does work.

Milk is very widely used for relief of nocturnal pain and you will hear many patients state that their standard remedy at home when wakened by symptoms is a glass of milk and a biscuit. It is of course no more effective than antacid preparation and excessive ingestion of milk is not to be encouraged as it will lead to the additional problem of obesity.

ANTISPASMODICS

These drugs are given the name antispasmodics because they act by relieving the muscle spasm of the stomach and duodenum which is found in ulcer patients. Smooth muscle in spasm for any length of time generates pain. If this spasm can be abolished many patients experience relief from their ulcer pain. The drugs which are used to do this, act by antagonising the action of acetylcholine on the parasympathetic nervous system and are therefore sometimes referred to as anticholinergic agents. You will remember that acetylcholine is the substance which transmits the nervous impulse from the parasympathetic nerves to the target organ. Anticholinergic drugs have no effect on the sympathetic nerves. The parasympathetic nervous system causes contraction of smooth muscle in the bowel and if its action is blocked by anticholinergic agents then the effect will be to cause relaxation of the smooth muscle of the bowel and to abolish spasm. The two most commonly used of these substances are atropine and propantheline.

Atropine

Atropine is administered orally in the form of atropine sulphate tablets. You may occasionally see the old fashioned tincture of belladona used, and belladona alkaloids are included in some proprietary antacids to produce an antispasmodic effect. Atropine is also available for intramuscular or intravenous administration and this is how it is most commonly used in hospital practice, being given routinely as premedication before surgery to dry up intestinal secretions. Atropine's ability to relax smooth muscle makes it valuable in the symptomatic relief of biliary and renal colic when severe pain results from muscle spasm in the bile duct or ureter. In these circumstances it is frequently given in combination with opiates as these drugs will actually increase smooth muscle spasm during the acute attack of pain.

Atropine, by virtue of its effect in blocking one effect of acetylcholine on the parasympathetic nervous system, has a variety of actions other than relief of smooth muscle spasm. It inhibits the secretions of salivary glands thus causing dryness of the mouth and also inhibits the bronchial secretions. For this reason it is often given preoperatively to lessen the risk of the patient inhaling salivary and bronchial secretions during anaesthesia. The drug is given in these circumstances by intramuscular injection in a dose of 0.6 mg.

Sweating is reduced in patients who receive atropine and because it inhibits the effect of the vagus nerve on the heart, the pulse usually quickens when the drug is administered. Blurring of vision also occurs with atropine and it may precipitate an attack of acute glaucoma in the elderly.

Propantheline

This drug has a similar action to atropine and is available as a tablet or as parenteral preparation. It is given in a dose of 15 or 30 mg orally or intramuscularly, and its side effects are very similar.

Method of administration of antispasmodics

A point which is not realised sufficiently often is that these drugs must be given *to the limit of the patient's tolerance* if they are to be effective. This means that the dose must be increased until the patient starts to complain of blurring of vision, dryness of the mouth or difficulty with micturition, these being the first symptoms of over-dosage with anticholinergic agents. When this stage is reached the dose is reduced to that which the patient can just tolerate without experiencing side effects. It is only at this level of dosage that one can hope to block the action of the parasympathetic nervous system on the smooth muscle of the bowel.

DRUGS WHICH HEAL ULCERS

Having informed you that antacids and antispasmodics are of little real help in influencing the healing of an ulcer you may ask if any drugs do. It has been known for a long time that cessation of smoking and enforced bed-rest both accelerate the healing process. The first remedy still holds true, and all patients with peptic ulcers should be constantly encouraged to give up the habit. Prolonged bed-rest of course is wasteful and has its own risks although even nowadays the patient with really severe symptoms may require a period of immobilisation. Much attention has been given in recent years to developing drugs which induce ulcer healing. Many claims have been made but at present there are only two groups of drugs for which there is convincing evidence of their efficacy. The two groups are the liquorice derivatives and the H^2 receptor antagonists.

The Liquorice derivatives

Carbenoxolone

This drug is extracted from the liquorice root, indeed liquorice extracts have been used as folk remedies for many years in the treatment of ulcer and with good effect. It has been known for several years that carbenoxolone promotes healing of gastric ulcers. Controversy has existed regarding its ability to heal duodenal ulcers but the advent of routine fiberoptic endoscopy has produced more accurate information, and there is now evidence that carbenoxolone is also effective in duodenal ulcer.

Dosage ranges from 50 to 100 mg thrice daily for periods of 4 to 6 weeks. Side effects are common, particularly in the elderly where the drug may cause fluid retention by the kidneys sufficient to precipitate congestive cardiac failure. Excessive urinary loss of potassium may also occur resulting extreme muscle weakness. Patients therefore should receive in-patient treatment with carbonoxolone or they should be seen once weekly as outpatients.

Glycyrrhizinic acid

This substance is contained in proprietary preparations which combine it with conventional antacids. It is derived from liquorice and is free of the side effects such as fluid retention and hypertension which accompany the use of carbenoxolone. Unfortunately it is also free of any healing effect and is really no better than standard antacids.

H^2 Receptor antagonists

Drugs which block histamine receptors in the stomach (see Ch. 1) are called histamine (H^2) receptor antagonists. When blockade occurs there is a marked reduction in gastric acid secretion and this will in time lead to ulcer healing. A number of compounds with this action were developed for experimental purposes but only one drug is currently in general use, cimetidine.

Cimetidine

Cimetidine was developed for treatment of duodenal ulcers and it will produce complete healing in a high proportion of cases. Later experience revealed that the drug is also effective in gastric ulcers, with approximately the same success rate as carbenoxolone but with freedom from the latter's common side effects, noted above. Cimetidine is therefore a better drug for treatment of gastric ulcer in the elderly. The main value of cimetidine, however, is in the treatment of duodenal ulcers. The usual dosage regime is 200 mg thrice daily and 400 mg at night. This is generally continued for about 6 to 8 weeks at which time healing of the ulcer has usually taken place. Thereafter the patient can be kept on a maintenance dose of 400 mg each night. The main drawback of this drug is that once treatment is discontinued the ulcer will reappear in a high proportion of cases. It does not seem to produce permanent healing and therefore cannot replace surgery as a cure. Although it is obviously going to be very valuable drug, the exact place of cimetidine in the overall management of duodenal ulcer is yet to be established.

THE PLACE OF DIET IN THE TREATMENT OF PEPTIC ULCER

There is no good evidence that strict diets contribute much to the management of peptic ulcer. In the past a bland diet consisting of fish paste, soft boiled eggs, mashed potatoes, semolina and other mouth-watering delicacies such as these was confidently prescribed in the rather naive belief that these foods would not irritate the ulcer and would allow it to heal. It has now been shown that such thinking was misguided. Your patient could live on milk and mashed potatoes for the rest of his days and this would have no effect on the healing of his ulcer. What advice then are you to give your ulcer patient concerning his diet? The answer can best be summed up in the following statement which you should make to your patient: 'It's *your* ulcer and *you* should learn how to live with it.' If he finds that eating curried foods gives him pain from his ulcer, he should obviously avoid curry. If this does not cause him pain he can eat as much of it as he wishes. If some ulcer patients develop pain after eating mashed potatoes, they should not eat mashed potatoes. Patients very quickly learn which foods they can and cannot eat without pain. It is wrong to prohibit certain foods because we feel they may irritate the stomach and prevent ulcer healing. There is no medical evidence that this is so. These remarks also apply to the consumption of alcohol. It is for your patient, not you, to decide whether alcohol is painful, or whether it has no effect on his ulcer.

There is one tenet about food which ulcer patients will find helpful. Small frequent meals rather than large infrequent ones will prevent pain. Food eaten every 2 hours or so will not help his ulcer heal but it will ward off attacks of pain by constantly neutralising acid in the stomach.

PURGATIVES

A wide selection of drugs with a purgative action is available to the nursing profession and to the lay public as across-the-counter sales. These drugs are misused by the public, the main reasons being a general obsession with bowel habit and widespread misunderstanding of what represents 'normal' bowel function.

In any aspect of the physiology of the human body there is a wide and acceptable variation from one person to another. This is as true of the bowel habits and the number of bowel motions passed per day as of anything else. Many people pass a bowel motion three times a day; this is not abnormal. Some pass a bowel motion once every three days; this is not abnormal. An *alteration* in the bowel habit *is* abnormal: for example, from one motion a day to one motion every three days. The remedy for this is *not* purgation but a medical examination and perhaps a Barium enema to ensure that no disease of the bowel, such as a neoplasm is present.

Continued purgation will reduce the tone of the intestinal musculature. Bowel function will then diminish and eventually a bowel motion will only occur when a purgative is given. Once this vicious circle is established it is very difficult to break. It is likely that misunderstanding about bowel function in general, and the need for purgatives in particular, extends into the nursing and medical profession. Purgatives certainly have a place in the management of established constipation, particularly in the elderly where poor diet may be a factor. The non-irritant purgatives are of value in the prevention of constipation in patients who are immobilised for a period, particularly when they also receive drugs which reduce intestinal motility, such as opiates.

Purgatives fall into four main groups. They are:

1. Bulk purgatives

2. Lubricant purgatives
3. Irritant purgatives
4. Miscellaneous.

Bulk purgatives

Bulk purgatives act by increasing the volume of intestinal content. By doing so they stimulate the large bowel to evacuate its contents. Magnesium sulphate is an example, and this drug increases intestinal contents by absorbing water and swelling. It produces fairly vigorous purgation and is still popular for the emergency purgation of the colon in hepatic coma when it is an advantage to remove excessive protein often in the form of altered blood from the gastrointestinal tract.

'Natural' bulk purgatives derived from bran or ispaghula husks are now very commonly used. Like magnesium sulphate they absorb water, swelling and stimulating peristalsis. In addition to their efficacy in constipation these drugs are now considered an important part of the management of the irritable bowel syndrome (spastic colon), diverticular disease and some cases of Crohn's disease and ulcerative colitis. These drugs are often supplied in the form of granules, which are taken with food.

Lubricant purgatives

As their name implies these act by lubricating the faeces. Liquid paraffin is a well known lubricant purgative. This substance should not be given for a long period of time but only on a short-term basis because tumours of the mediastinal lymph nodes may develop in patients who have been taking liquid paraffin for a number of years. Liquid paraffin also interferes with the absorption of fat soluble vitamins (A, D, K).

Irritant purgatives

These act locally on the large bowel, and stimulate the evacuation of its contents. The most famous of the group is the foul-tasting castor oil which acts from 2 to 6 hours after ingestion. This should not be used nowadays. Perhaps the most popular agent in this group is senna. The active principle in this drug is a substance known as emodin. Emodin is one of a group of agents known as anthraquinones. Cascara is another well known drug which also contains emodin. This chemical requires to be absorbed into the blood stream before it can be active. It stimulates contraction of smooth muscle in the colon and its purgative action is often accompanied by colicky pains.

Miscellaneous purgatives

These include a group of purgatives with variable actions on the bowel. Perhaps the most interesting is the drug phenolphthalein which is a mild purgative and is the active ingredient of a large number of proprietary purgatives. This drug is used by inorganic chemists as an indicator in acid-alkali titrations. It turns red in alkaline solutions and is colourless in acid solutions. If a patient taking phenolphthalein excretes an acid urine therefore, all is well. If, however, he excretes an alkaline urine, a red colour is observed. This can be alarming to the patient and the nurse alike. It is therefore worth remembering about phenolphthalein. Another interesting side effect is that the drug occasionally gives rise to a fixed drug eruption. When some patients take the drug they develop a red blotchy rash which disappears when the drug is stopped. If they start to take phenolphthalein again, however, the rash comes back in exactly the same place.

Suppositories

Suppositories exert their action in producing purgation by a direct irritant effect locally on the rectal mucosa. You should advise your patient not to expect an immediate result after inserting a suppository. It must be retained in the rectum for a sufficient length of time for the body temperature to melt the gelatinous base and release the drug so that it may then act locally. Bisacodyl (Dulcolax) suppositories both stimulate and lubricate the rectum. They are especially valuable in the management of constipation in the elderly bedridden patient provided there is no impacted faeces in the rectum.

Glycerin suppositories have a weaker action than bisacodyl suppositories. They are of great value, however, in the treatment of haemorrhoids because they lubricate the rectum in such a way as to prevent the patient straining and causing painful prolapse of his haemorrhoids.

Enemata

These work as bulk prugatives by distending the rectal and colonic mucosa. A commonly used enema consists of soft soap (1 oz) made up to 20 fl ozs with water. This mixture is insufflated into the rectum after being gently warmed to prevent unnecessary discomfort to the patient. Disposable enemata are now used in most hospitals.

Enemata are employed to remove impacted faeces from the rectum where a suppository has failed. They are often used in patients confined to bed for a long time or in the elderly. In both of these situations the muscles of the bowel become sluggish. Enemata are also used to empty the large bowel prior to radiological examination of the alimentary tract, the gallbladder or the kidneys and before some surgical operations on the intestines. Another reason for using enemata is to bring a drug into contact with the rectal and colonic mucosa. This is most commonly one of the steroid drugs which are used in the management of ulcerative colitis (see below).

DRUGS WHICH CONTROL DIARRHOEA

Clearly, the correct approach to diarrhoea is to find the cause and treat it. However, sometimes by reason of severity of the patient's complaint it is desirable to treat the diarrhoea symptomatically while specific treatment takes effect. Alternatively, it may be that there is no specific treatment for the diarrhoea and symptomatic treatment is all that can be 'offered'. A number of drugs are useful in the symptomatic treatment of diarrhoea. Both morphine and codeine diminish the propulsive activity of the large and the small bowel. Codeine is to be preferred to morphine because of the danger of producing addiction to morphine. It is usually administered in the form of codeine phosphate tablets, given as a dose of 30–60 mg three of four times daily. If the patient is unlikely to recover from his illness, however (for example, if his diarrhoea is due to inoperable carcinoma of the large bowel) then morphine is the better drug as it is more potent than codeine. These substances are often administered with either chalk or kaolin both of which have strong water-absorbing properties and both of which therefore contribute to the control of the diarrhoea by making the stool more formed. A typical preparation is chalk and opium mixture where the active ingredient of the opium is morphine.

Newer drugs such as diphenoxylate (Lomotil) and loperamide are now widely used for the symptomatic treatment of diarrhoea. They are chemically related to the opiates but are free of the analgesic and addictive effects. They inhibit smooth muscle activity in the bowel and can be of help in the treatment of diarrhoea resulting from a wide variety of disease processes.

DRUGS USED IN THE TREATMENT OF INFLAMMATORY BOWEL DISEASE

The term inflammatory bowel disease covers two important entities in the United Kingdom—ulcerative colitis and Crohn's disease. Although there are differences between these conditions there are also many similarities. Whereas Crohn's disease can produce extensive damage to the small intestine, ulcerative colitis is always confined to the large bowel. However, when Crohn's disease affects the colon and rectum the two conditions can be difficult to distinguish and as the treatment is virtually the same we shall consider them together. When a new patient presents with acute inflammation in the colon there are two distinct phases to his management. The first step is to induce a remission and the second is to maintain this remission indefinitely.

Corticosteroids

Corticosteroids are the drugs of choice in suppressing acute colitis. In the severe case they are usually administered orally or intravenously. When the oral route is chosen prednisolone is the most popular drug and this is given in a dose of 40 to 80 mg per day, the dose being reduced once the condition starts to come under control. In less severe cases, when the disease is confined to the rectum with sparing of the rest of the large bowel, prednisolone or hydrocortisone can be administered by enemata. In this situation the drug acts partly by a local effect on the rectal mucosa and partly by being absorbed into the blood stream through the rectal mucosa. Corticosteroids will produce a remission in the majority of patients with acute colitis but they are not very effective in preventing further relapses. For this reason patients with inflammatory bowel disease are seldom left on corticosteroids indefinitely. They are of course still subject to the common and serious side effects which are associated with the use of these drugs and are discussed in detail in Chapter 8.

Sulphasalazine

This is an unusual drug, being a combination of a sulphonamide and salicylic acid. Why it is effective in colitis is not clearly understood. Although it is of little value in the acute phase of the disease it is much more effective than steroids in preventing further relapses of the condition. When used in doses of 2 g or more per day it will maintain a remission indefinitely in a large proportion of patients with ulcerative colitis. Side effects are quite common with sulphasalazine, particularly if high doses are used for any length of time. Nausea is a common complaint and more serious adverse reactions include renal damage and haemolytic anaemia. The side effects of sulphonamides are discussed in more detail in the chapter on antibacterial agents.

While Crohn's disease affecting the large bowel will often respond to the treatment outlined above, although not as well as ulcerative colitis, inflammation of the small intestine which is often extensive in this condition usually proves resistant to medical treatment. At present there is no really effective therapy for this distressing condition.

DRUGS USED IN DISORDERS OF THE LIVER

In general there are no specific drug remedies for diseases which affect the liver. The management of the patient with a hepatic disorder is determined by its cause.

A gallstone impacted in a bile duct clearly requires surgical removal whereas the patient with acute hepatitis requires general medical care. The treatment of acute liver failure from any cause is a specialised subject and discussion is outwith the scope of this book.

Cholestyramine

This drug binds bile acids in the intestine after oral administration. The bound bile acids cannot be reabsorbed and are excreted in the faeces.

Bile acids cause severe itching of the skin in patients with biliary obstruction. If the obstruction to the flow of bile acids from the liver to the duodenum is *complete* cholestyramine is ineffectual as there are no bile acids in the bowel which can be bound and thereafter excreted. If the biliary obstruction is *partial* however (that is if some bile acids are entering the duodenum) then the drug prevents the reabsorption of these and consequently lowers bile acid levels in the plasma. Consequently cholestyramine relieves pruritus in some patients with partial biliary obstruction.

The drug is also of value in the treatment of diarrhoea occurring in patients following ileal resection. Here bile salts which are normally reabsorbed in the ileum pass to the colon where they have a purgative effect. By binding these salts cholestyramine reduces the diarrhoea.

The dose of cholestyramine varies from 4 to 12 g daily.

Chenodeoxycholic acid

This is a new drug which has been shown to have the ability to dissolve gallstones. Most gallstones are formed of cholesterol and this drug by lowering the concentration of cholesterol in the bile causes them to slowly dissolve. It will only work in the presence of a functioning gall-bladder and is ineffective against calcified gallstones. It should only be used under hospital supervision and after appropriate radiological investigation. Patients require to be treated with the drug for a long time and as liver damage can sometimes occur as a side effect the liver function tests are monitored during therapy.

DRUGS USED IN DISORDERS OF THE PANCREAS

As in liver disease, there are no really effective drugs for the management of pancreatic disorders. Patients suffering from acute pancreatitis may be very ill and successful management depends on good supportive care.

Aprotinin (Trasylol)

This drug has been available for several years and evidence as to its success in the treatment of acute pancreatitis has been conflicting. If there is any benefit to be gained from its use it is probably very slight. The drug's action is to inhibit protease enzymes which are liberated into the abdominal cavity and blood stream in high concentrations during an attack of pancreatitis. Aprotinin is administered by constant intravenous infusion.

Pancreatin

The pancreas has two main functions both of which may fail if the gland is extensively damaged by disease or removed at operation. The endocrine function is the production of insulin and this is discussed in Chapter 11. The exocrine function is the production of digestive ensymes such as lipase and amylase. When secretion of these enzymes is deficient, oral replacement therapy is given. Pancreatin is an extract of animal (beef or hog) pancreas containing to a variable extent pancreatic enzymes concerned with the digestion and breakdown of proteins, fats and starches.

The uses of pancreatin are mainly in the treatment of children with cystic fibrosis of the pancreas. These children have deficient secretion of the pancreatic digestive enzymes and treatment with pancreatin improves the absorption of fats and protein and reduces diarrhoea which is often a distressing feature of cystic fibrosis. The drug is also given to patients with chronic pancreatitis or some individuals following certain types of gastric surgery.

The most effective way to administer pancreatin is as a powder scattered on food, but it has a very unpleasant taste and children find it objectionable. It can therefore be given immediately before meals dissolved in *cold* sweetened milk or fruit juice. Because the enzymes in pancreatin are inactivated by heat, the powder should not be dissolved in hot drinks nor should it be taken with very hot foods. The actions of these enzymes are also inactivated by hydrochloric acid. This is very inconvenient as much of the drug's activity is therefore lost in the stomach. The discovery of the H^2 receptor antagonist drug cimetidine has allowed us to block the secretion of gastric acid in these patients and cimetidine is now frequently given along with pancreatin, greatly increasing the benefit of this drug.

Occasionally pancreatic extracts can burn the buccal mucosa and the skin round the mouth of the anus. A barrier cream affords some protection against this. Some patients develop sensitivity reactions to the powder; these are manifested by sneezing, skin reactions and asthma.

3

Drugs used in the treatment of diseases of the heart and circulation

DRUGS USED TO TREAT CARDIAC FAILURE

Digitalis

Digitalis was first introduced into clinical practice by the English physician William Withering in 1785. Withering noticed that some of his patients with dropsy (oedema) became much improved following the ingestion of a remedy given them by a local herablist. He investigated this remedy and found that the active ingredient came from the leaf of the dried foxglove and he accordingly named the new treatment for dropsy 'digitalis' (Digitalis is the Latin word for foxglove).

There are two main kinds of preparations in common use:

1. Digitoxin.
2. Digoxin.

The substance digitalis is not a chemically pure one as it contains traces of other chemicals which are pharmacologically inert. As the drug is standardised using a bio-assay procedure, variation in strength between different batches of digitalis is to be expected and is indeed found. For this reason the chemically pure substance digoxin is to be preferred to digitalis. Digitoxin is also chemically pure as it is purified from digitalis. Most physicians in Great Britain treat their patients with digoxin and this is therefore the preparation which you will see used most commonly in the wards and with which you should be completely familiar.

Physiology of the heart. Before discussing the actions of digoxin a brief resume of some aspects of the physiology of the heart pertinent to this topic seems appropriate. You will recall that the heart has an inherent power of contraction and that this power resides in the cardiac muscle fibres. If the heart is isolated from a living subject and all nerves to it are cut, rhythmic contractions will be observed for the period before the cardiac muscle dies. The way in which the contraction is propagated rhythmically throughout the heart is illustrated in Figure 3.1. An electrical impulse starts in the sino-atrial node high on the wall of the right atrium. This impulse spreads throughout the entire wall of the right atrium and then the left atrium, and as it does so it stimulates the atrial muscle to contract. The impulse then reaches the atrio-ventricular node, a specialised tissue which has the property of rapidly conducting electrical impulses of this sort. The impulse therefore rapidly descends through the atrio-ventricular node to the bundle of His which is composed of the same sort of tissue as the node. As Figure 3.1 shows, the bundle of His runs down both sides of the interventricular septum and spreads up the sides of the right and left ventricles. From this bundle little twigs of specialised electrical-conducting tissue run deep into the walls of the ventricles carrying the impulse which stimulates the ventricular muscle to contract. It is important to appreciate that in normal health (when the heart rate is 70 to 90 beats per minute) each time the atria contract, an electrical message is sent down the bundle of His to the ventricles and they then contract, ensuring that blood which the atria have pumped into them is in turn pumped into the pulmonary artery and the aorta.

In the condition atrial fibrillation the atria contract at a rate of approximately 600 beats per minute. In fact at such a high rate there are no real contractions and the atria merely quiver unable to pump blood properly into the ventricles. Enough blood drains through the atria into the ventricles to maintain the circulation, but life would not continue if each of these electrical impulses was conducted into the ventricles resulting in a rate of 600 beats per minute. The bundle of His and atrio-ventricular

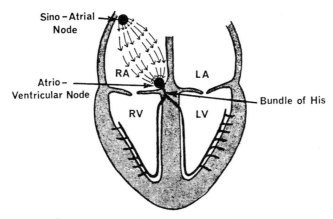

Fig. 3.1. The spread of the impulse which originates in the pace-maker in the sino-atrial node through the cardiac muscle is shown.

node do their best to rectify matters by transmitting only every third, fourth, fifth and sixth beat in an irregular fashion, and by refusing to transmit the beats in between. This manoeuvre is partially successful in slowing the pulse so that the rate in untreated patients with atrial fibrillation is usually between 100 and 200 beats per minute and the rhythm is irregular. Such a heart rate is still unsatisfactory if it persists for any length of time because it is extremely tiring for the heart muscle. One of the main actions of digoxin is to remedy the fast ventricular heart rate which occurs in untreated atrial fibrillation.

Actions of digoxin. Digoxin has a variety of actions. The three main ones are:

1. It increases the power of contraction of the heart muscle
2. It prolongs the period during which the bundle of His cannot transmit a contraction
3. It increases the excitability of the heart muscle.

The first two of these actions explain many of the therapeutic uses of digoxin. The third accounts for some of the very dangerous side effects of this drug.

Digoxin increases the power of heart muscle contraction. In congestive cardiac failure the muscular power of the heart is not sufficient for the job of pumping blood round the circulation. The backlog of blood which the heart has failed to pump simultaneously into the aorta and pulmonary artery piles up in the veins. When this happens the pressure of blood in the veins rises and fluid is therefore pushed out of them into the tissues. You will see evidence of this in your patient with congestive cardiac failure as sacral and leg oedema, distension of the veins of the neck and dyspnoea with white frothy spit. This last is due to engorgement of the pulmonary veins which leads to transudation of fluid into the alveoli of the lung.

Digoxin is especially good at improving the contractile power of heart muscle which is failing at its job although how it actually does this is not known. There are two effects which stem from digoxin-induced improvement in cardiac muscular contraction.

1. The backlog of blood which the heart should have pumped into the aorta and pulmonary artery is cleared away. You will often see that this lessens the distension in the neck veins and causes an improvement in your patient's breathing and in his sacral and leg oedema.

2. The second effect of increasing the power of cardiac muscular contraction is that the blood is driven more forcibly to the organs and tissues. The improvement in blood flow to the kidneys is particularly noticeable and digoxin on its own may produce a diuresis in patients with cardiac failure. In practice of course diuretic drugs are usually prescribed with digoxin in this situation.

Digoxin prolongs the period during which the bundle of His cannot transmit a contraction. This action is responsible for the beneficial effects of digoxin in patients with atrial fibrillation. As has been previously discussed, in patients with this condition the bundle of His tries to slow the heart rate by irregularly transmitting only some of the impulses reaching it from the atria. It is, however, only partially successful in this attempt and fast heart rates are the rule in untreated atrial fibrillation. By prolonging the period during which the bundle of His is refractory to stimulation by electrical impulses coming from the atria, digoxin can slow the number of impulses transmitted by the bundle to the ventricles and can thus slow the ventricular rate. This is of immense benefit to the heart, because when the ventricle is beating very fast (say at 180 beats per minute) there is hardly any time between beats for it to fill with blood. This means that many of the ventricular beats may cause virtually no blood to be ejected. The heart muscle is therefore clearly working grossly inefficiently. When the ventricular rate is slowed through the action of digoxin on the bundle of His, the situation is vastly improved: there is time for the ventricles to fill with blood between each beat and consequently the heart works much more efficiently in terms of the amounts of blood ejected for the amount of work done by the heart muscle.

You will have noticed that digoxin does not alter the atrial rate in atrial fibrillation: this continues to be approximately 600 beats per minute. Moreover, although the number of impulses transmitted by the bundle of His is reduced by digoxin therapy, such impulses as are transmitted reach the ventricles irregularly. The pulse of the patient remains irregular but is slower whereas before treatment it was irregular and fast.

Digoxin increases the excitability of the heart muscle. This action of digoxin is a very important one for it is responsible for the serious side effects of the drug. Multiple extrasystoles, ventricular tachycardia and ventricular fibrillation are all produced by the excitative or irritant effect which digoxin has on cardiac muscle. These potentially fatal conditions fortunately occur only when an *overdose* of digoxin has been given and premonitory signs and symptoms of them are always present. The nature of the warning signs of digoxin overdosage and the side effects of the drug are discussed later.

Principles of administration of digoxin.

It is vital that you have a clear grasp of the principles observed in digitalising a patient. Trying to digitalise a patient is rather like trying to fill a bath tub full of water with the bath-plug left out! If you were to run water into such a bath as a slow trickle you would fill it only after a very long time, perhaps never. The obvious thing to do in such a situation would be to run the bath taps very briskly so that what goes into the bath more than compensates for what is running out of the plug-hole. As soon as the bath is full, however, you must maintain the water at the level you want by cutting down on the water going in so that it just balances the water going out.

You may feel this is a very inefficient way to run a bath but when it comes to digitalising the patient this is more or less the procedure one must adopt. Patients excrete digoxin mainly in the urine and in this respect they resemble the bath with the plug left out. In order to achieve a therapeutic concentration of digoxin a large loading dose of digoxin must be given (equivalent to running both taps briskly) and then the dose must be reduced to a maintenance dose (equivalent to maintaining the water at a constant level in the bath) otherwise the patient will develop symptoms of digoxin intoxication (equivalent to the water in the bath running over!).

Now just as there are various sizes of baths and various speeds you could fill them at (depending on precisely how briskly you run the taps in the beginning) so patients have differing requirements for digoxin to become fully digitalised. Each clinical situation requires individual assessment. However, for all patients and in all situations the principle is the same: a large digitalising dose followed by a smaller maintenance dose of digoxin. In practice this loading dose is usually given over a period of a day, for instance 0.25 mg 6 hourly for 24 hours or 0.25 mg 8 hourly for 24 hours. In some centres the patients are given one single digitalizing dose of say 0.75 to 1.0 mg. No further drug is given for 24 hours and the patients are then started on their daily maintenance dose of, say, 0.25 mg. This second method seems to work just as well. The loading dose of digoxin is mainly determined by the patient's size. A large man requires a higher dose to fill the various body compartments than a small woman. On the other hand the maintenance dose of digoxin is determined by the kidney function (analogous to the size of the plughole in the bath referred to above). Patients with reduced renal function (particularly in old age) require a reduced maintenance dose and patients in advanced renal failure require a very small dose indeed. Some people attempt to calculate a dose of digoxin for each patient separately from a formula which takes into account such factors as age, body weight and renal function. It has been possible using this method to reduce the toxicity from digoxin as well as improving the effect. An interesting fact which emerged from this is that some patients need unusual doses of digoxin, for instance 0.125 mg, 0.1875 mg or 0.375 mg per day, instead of the customary 0.25 or 0.5 mg per day which were the doses most commonly used in the past. The old habit of simply giving digoxin until signs of toxicity appear before reducing the dose is no longer recommended.

Symptoms and signs of digoxin toxicity.

The manifestations of digoxin toxicity can occur at any time but commonly appear between the second and fifth day of treatment. As the patient complains first to the nurses it is important that the nurse is well acquainted with this subject.
The side effects are:

1. Anorexia, nausea and vomiting
2. Headache, fatigue and drowsiness
3. Irregularities of the rate and rhythm of the heart. (These are important because they can lead to death of the patient)
4. Disorientation and confusion in old people.

Many drugs cause anorexia, nausea and vomiting when given orally but it is particularly important to recognise that in a patient on digoxin therapy these symptoms may be the first signs of digoxin intoxication. Anorexia occurring in such a patient is a clear indiciation for stopping treatment with digoxin until the symptom improves. When this happens treatment is restarted in a lower dose. Digoxin intoxication can occur quite suddenly even although the patient has been taking the drug for years in a balanced maintenance dose.
  Patients on digoxin therapy sometimes complain of headache or drowsiness and this too may be an early sign of digoxin intoxication. The complaint, however, occurs very much less often than anorexia which is the symptom for which you must be on the lookout.
  The side effects of digoxin on the heart are numerous. Any irregularity of rhythm or rate may occur. Therefore any change which you observe when you take the pulse of your patient on digoxin therapy is worthwhile reporting to a senior colleague. The change you have detected may necessitate stopping the drug for a while. Never be ashamed to ask a colleague for advice in this situation if you are in doubt about the rate or rhythm of the pulse. The most commonly occurring abnormalities in the heart due to overdosage of this drug are:

1. Bradycardia
2. Ventricular extrasystoles
3. Coupling
4. Tachycardia due to ventricular tachycardia.

Bradycardia is excessive slowing of the heart and comes about through the action of digoxin on the atrio-ventricular node. If a pulse of 60 or less beats per minute is recorded this is an indication for stopping digoxin therapy until the pulse rises above this figure and then restarting the drug usually in a smaller dose. The other three abormalities, ventricular extrasystoles, coupling and ventricular tachycardia are all manifestations of the effect which digoxin has in increasing the excitability of the heart muscle. A few ventricular extrasystoles occur in healthy people from time to time but regularly occurring extrasystoles in a patient on digoxin are a warning sign of overdosage. A curious and interesting form of extrasystole is sometimes observed in these patients. Each normal beat of the heart is followed immediately by an extrasystole. A long pause then ensues before the cycles of normal beat-extrasystole repeats itself. This sequence is known as 'coupling' of the heart beat and it is easily appreciated when you take the pulse at the wrist. To help you remember about coupling, the phenomenon is illustrated in Figure 3.2. which shows the electrocardiographic tracing taken from a patient with coupling of the pulse. The normal beat is immediately followed by a beat with an abnormal shape on the electrocardiogram. This is the ventricular extrasystole giving rise to the coupling of the pulse which was felt at this patient's wrist.

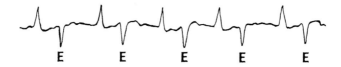

E   E   E   E   E

Fig. 3.2. The electrocardiographic tracing of the heart in a patient with coupling of the pulse. The letter E refers to the abnormal ventricular beat which follows each normal beat (unmarked).

If one were to ignore all the premonitory signs of digoxin intoxication and one continued to give the patient digoxin he would eventually develop the grave condition of ventricular *tachycardia* which could lead to death. Sometimes the ventricles, instead of beating too fast, start to *fibrillate*. In this case the shimmering movements of the muscle of the ventricular wall are totally inadequate to eject any blood out of the heart and death ensues in a matter of *minutes*. Death from digoxin overdosage is a preventable condition. It should never occur, yet every year a number of people die due to the toxic effects of this drug. It often happens that patients being treated with digoxin are also receiving diuretic therapy (for example, patients with congestive cardiac failure). A side effect of diuretic therapy is loss of the electrolyte, potassium. Patients who are potassium-depleted are especially liable to digoxin intoxication. Always be especially on your guard therefore when a patient on digoxin and diuretic treatment complains of anorexia or exhibits a slow or coupled pulse.

Elderly patients are liable occasionally to disorientation due to the effects of digoxin and one occasionally sees patients who become quite maniacal on this drug (the so-called 'digoxin-madness'). This is, you will be relieved to learn, a rare condition.

Nursing observations on patients being treated with digoxin

Much of this follows from the discussion of the side effects and the actions of digoxin.

1. Watch for the development of anorexia, nausea and vomiting.

2. Watch for the development of a slow or a coupled pulse or the development of any irregularity which was not previously noted. It is customary in many hospitals for the nurse giving medicines to take the patient's pulse before giving digoxin. If the pulse is below 60 the dose is withheld and a report given to sister.

3. In patients who are being treated with digoxin for atrial fibrillation you should record the pulse rate at the wrist and the ventricular heart rate at the apex. The difference between these two is known as the *pulse deficit*. This is a measure of the number of weak ventricular beats which are not strong enough to be felt at the wrist. In normal health or in well-controlled atrial fibrillation the pulse deficit is zero. The higher the pulse deficit the less well-controlled is the fibrillation because a high pulse deficit means that the left ventricle is beating so quickly and irregularly that it is having little time to fill up with blood between some beats. These beats are therefore not expelling sufficient blood to be felt as a pulse at the wrist. Figure 3.3 shows the wrist and apex rate of a patient who was treated with digoxin for a very fast atrial fibrillation. Notice how the pulse deficit decreased and the heart rate slowed as he was brought under control with digoxin.

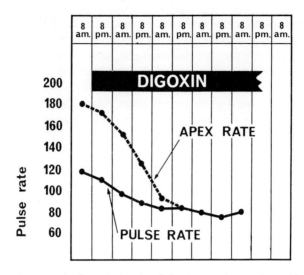

Fig. 3.3. Decrease in the apical and radial pulse rate in a patient with atrial fibrillation during treatment with digoxin.

4. A measure of the volume of the patient's daily urinary output should be kept if digoxin is being given for the treatment of congestive cardiac failure. This can be conveniently done by recording details of the amount of urine excreted and the amount of fluid ingested on a fluid balance chart. Fluid balance charts are discussed on p. 48.

Uses of digoxin

The main uses of digoxin are in the treatment of:

1. Congestive cardiac failure and left ventricular failure
2. Atrial fibrillation and other supraventricular tachycardias.

In heart failure usually both sides of the heart fail at the same time. Occasionally a single ventricle (left or right) is the main side to fail and left ventricular failure responds well to digoxin.

Atrial fibrillation is called a supraventricular tachycardia because the fast heart rate arises in the atria above (supra) the ventricles. There are other tachycardias which occasionally arise in the atria as when the atria beat very fast rather than fibrillate. These supraventricular tachycardias respond well to digoxin. Here the action of the drug is virtually the same as in atrial fibrillation (see digoxin in the treatment of cardiac arrhythmics p. 49).

Diuretics

A diuretic is a substance which increases the flow of urine. In practice this means increasing the secretion of water and sodium by the kidney. Many substances have been used in the past to increase the flow of urine in patients suffering from cardiac failure and other diseases which cause oedema. Most of these substances are now of historical interest because modern diuretics have made them obsolete. We now have access to a number of very potent and comparatively safe diuretic drugs which have revolutionised the treatment of cardiac failure, particularly in its most sudden and life threatening form: acute left ventricular failure.

SOME ASPECTS OF RENAL PHYSIOLOGY

Before discussing the action of the diuretics which are used in clinical practice, a brief recapitulation of those aspects of the physiology of the kidney necessary to the understanding of the

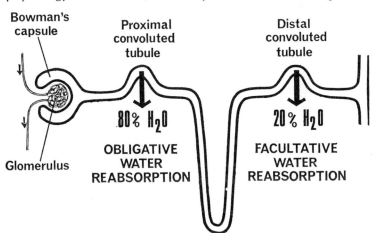

Fig. 3.4. Diagram of renal glomerulus and tubules (simplified). Approximately 80 per cent of the water filtered at the glomerulus is reabsorbed by the proximal convoluted tubules and 20 per cent by the distal tubules. The loop of Henle joins the proximal and distal convoluted tubules.

mode of action of these drugs may be helpful. Figure 3.4 shows a simplified diagram of the renal glomerulus and tubules. You will remember that blood enters the glomerular tuft via the afferent arteriole and leaves via the efferent arteriole. Fluid filters from the blood in the glomerular tuft across Bowman's capsule into the lumen of the kidney tubule. This fluid, which contains most of the electrolytes and substances found in plasma, first passes down the proximal tubule of the kidney. Here many substances are reabsorbed by the cells which line the kidney tubule. In particular, a great deal of water is reabsorbed. If this were not so then most of the great volume of water which passes from the glomerular tuft into the kidney tubule would be excreted and we should all have little time left for anything else but passing urine. The reabsorption of water from the lumen of the kidney tubule back into the tubule cell (and thence into the body) is referred to as 'obligative water reabsorption'. The term 'obligative' means that the kidney is *obliged* to reabsorb most of the water passing down this tubule. About 80 per cent of the water which filters from the glomerular tuft into the renal tubule is reabsorbed by obligative water reabsorption. The fluid still remaining in the proximal tubule of the kidney which has not been absorbed then passes down the loop of Henle where sodium is reabsorbed.

In the distal tubule of the kidney the electrolytes sodium ($Na+$) potassium ($K+$) and chloride (Cl) are reabsorbed. Now the kidney cannot reabsorb these substances in the solid form, they must be first dissolved in water. This means that when $Na+$, $K+$ or Cl are reabsorbed, water is also reabsorbed. The kidney has the power to vary the individual amounts of $Na+$, $K+$ and Cl reabsorbed according to the needs of the body at any given time. It thus has the faculty of controlling the amount of water reabsorbed in the distal tubule. The process of handling water in the distal tubule is therefore referred to as 'facultative' water reabsorption and this process accounts for about 20 per cent of the water filtered at the glomerulus.

The thiazide diuretics

These comprise a large family of chemically related substances (the benzo thiadiazines) These drugs differ from each other only in respect of their duration of action and dosage. They are given orally and act mainly on the distal tabule causing an increase in sodium and water secretion by the kidney. The thiadiazines in current use include *chlorothiazide* (dose 1 g), *hydrochlorothiazide* (100 mg), *hydroflumethiazide* (100 mg) and *bendrofluazide* (10 mg) all of which have a duration of action of about 12 hours. *Chlorthalidone* (100 mg), and *polythiazide* (1 mg) act for about 18 to 24 hours. Thiazide diuretics are usually given as a single morning dose. The diuretic action in most people is prolonged and fairly gentle so their main use is in the treatment of mild cardiac failure. These drugs also have a hypotensive effect and they are used as antihypertensive drugs (see section on treatment of hypertension).

Unwanted effects

Thiazide diuretics are extensively used and serious side effects are rare. All diuretic drugs may lead to dehydration and sodium deficiency and in this respect thiazides are no exception. Elderly patients are particularly at risk.

When a patient is given a thiazide diuretic there is an increased loss of potassium in the urine. Frequently there is a moderate fall in the plasma potassium concentration and occasionally this can be marked. This fact has led to widespread prescription of potassium supplements for patients receiving these drugs. In fact relatively few patients develop severe potassium deficiency and in practice it has been found that those with serious cardiac and hepatic failure are most at risk. Other groups of patients, in particular those receiving thiazides for treatment of hypertension, do not require regular potassium supplementation. It is of course a wise precaution to check the plasma potassium concentration from time to time once therapy has been started.

Thiazide diuretics have an effect on carbohydrate metabolism and patients with latent tendency to diabetes may develop a full-blown disease during therapy. These drugs also cause the body to retain uric acid and this occasionally leads to an attack of acute gout. Finally skin rashes may occur and very rarely there may be a reversible fall in the blood platelet count during treatment. This is known as thrombocytopenia.

Frusemide

This very valuable drug is chemically rather similar to the thiadiazine group of diuretics, but differs from these drugs in that it is a more potent diuretic agent and has a much more rapid onset of action. Frusemide acts mainly on the loop of Henle and produces loss of water Na+ and K+. The drug produces a diuresis within half an hour of oral administration and its duration of action is approximately 6 hours. When there is an urgent need for treatment as in acute left ventricular failure, frusemide will produce a diuresis with dramatic clinical improvement within 20 minutes if it is given intravenously. Another advantage of frusemide compared with thiazide diuretics is that it acts in situations where they may fail to produce a response such as in renal failure or in some patients in gross congestive cardiac failure or with ascites due to liver disease or the nephrotic syndrome.

A typical dose is 40 mg daily but in renal failure doses of the order of 0.5 to 1 g may be given. It is wise to give frusemide in the morning rather than in the evening where the drug may continue to act during the early hours of sleep thus causing inconvenience to the patient.

Unwanted effects

Like the thiazides, frusemide may lead to excessive loss of water and sodium ions with resulting hypotension. In fact this hazard is greater with frusemide because it is a much more potent drug. Old people are particularly at risk and must be observed carefully for this complication.

Potassium depletion may occur and is most likely during initial therapy when a very marked diuresis may occur, particularly in the oedematous patient. Potassium supplementation is necessary in this situation, particularly if the patient is also receiving digoxin, as hypokalaemia increases the risk of digoxin toxicity. Once the patient is free of oedema it is often possible to discontinue potassium supplements without incurring risk of serious deficiency.

As with thiazides, gout, diabetes mellitus, skin rashes and, rarely, thrombocytopenia can occur during frusemide therapy. When the drug is used in very high doses there is a risk of causing deafness. Finally, there is a very real risk of producing a urinary retention following a brisk diuresis. Again this is commoner in the elderly and should always be considered if the patient fails to pass urine after receiving the dose of a diuretic.

Bumetanide

This is a relatively new diuretic whose action is very similar to frusemide. On a weight to weight basis it is more potent than the older drug and is usually given in a dose of 0.5 to 1.0 mg. It is used in a similar fashion to frusemide and may be given intravenously in acute left ventricular failure when it has a very rapid onset of action. The side effects of bumetanide are not as well known as frusemide as it has not been in use for such a long time. They are likely to be very similar to the older drug.

Ethacrynic acid

This is a very potent diuretic with an action similar to frusemide. It may be given orally or intraveneously but its toxicity seems to be greater than that of frusemide with transient deafness and renal failure being reported as possible adverse effects. It is therefore used less frequently than the other diuretics mentioned in this section.

POTASSIUM SPARING DIURETICS

These drugs cause a retention of potassium by the body rather than a loss as is the case with the other diuretics. They are not very powerful agents and are usually used in conjunction with the thiadiazines, frusemide or ethacrynic acid. The potassium sparing diuretics are spironolactone, triamterene and amiloride.

Spironolactone

This diuretic has an interesting mechanism of action. In certain conditions associated with oedema, notably liver cirrhosis and nephrotic syndrome, and some cases of congestive cardiac failure, the adrenal gland is stimulated to secrete excess amounts of the powerful hormone aldosterone. The action of this substance is to cause the distal tubules of the kidney to reabsorb Na+ thus conserving the electrolyte in the body. As you might expect, when Na+ is reabsorbed, water is reabsorbed with it. The net action of aldosterone is therefore to cause excess retention of water and this in turn promotes the retention of oedema fluid even although the patient may be receiving diuretic therapy.

The effect of spironolactone is to block the action of aldosterone on the renal tubules and to allow the excretion of Na+ and water to take place. In this respect it acts as a competitive antagonist of aldosterone (see Mode of Action of Drugs). Some patients with oedema which is resistant to other forms of diuretic therapy respond dramatically when spironolactone is added to their regimen of treatment. Spironolactone has a slow onset of action and may take over a week to be effective. It is usually given in conjunction with other potent diuretics but may be used alone, particularly in cirrhosis with ascites when there are very high levels of aldosterone present in the blood.

Unwanted effects

Because of its steroid structure, spironolactone can have an oestrogen-like action and lead to breast development (gynecomastia) in the male. This is often painful. Because of its action in antagonising aldosterone, spironolactone may lead to excessive accumulation of potassium in the body. This is a very dangerous situation as hyperkalaemia (high plasma potassium concentration) can result in cardiac arrest. Potassium retention is a particular hazard in the elderly and those with impaired renal function.

Triamterene and amiloride

Triamterene and amiloride are chemically related substances which have a very weak diuretic action but are used because they tend to promote potassium retention. Their action is different from spironolactone in that they do not antagonise the effect of aldosterone. These drugs are often used in combination with thiazide diuretic and some proprietary preparations contain both in one tablet. Their main side effect is a tendency to promote potassium retention by the body and like spironolactone this is more likely in the presence of renal failure and in the elderly.

The uses of diuretics

Diuretics usually are used to treat oedema. Because these drugs increase the amount of fluid excreted by the kidney, the volume

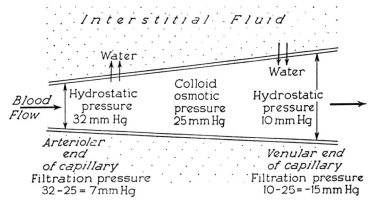

Fig. 3.5. At the arteriolar end of the capillary the hydrostatic pressure (blood pressure), which forces fluid *out* of the capillary, is about 32mm mercury. This pressure just exceeds the water holding effect of the albumin molecules (colloid osmotic pressure) which holds fluid *in* the capillary (25mm mercury). The net effect is that fluid tends to be pushed out of the arteriolar end of the capillary. At the venular end the hydrostatic effect of the blood pressure is much less than at the arteriolar end (about 10mm mercury). Consequently in normal health the colloid osmotic pressure exerted by the albumin molecules exceeds the hydrostatic pressure at the venular end of the capillary and water is sucked in.

In congestive cardiac failure, the back-log of blood in the veins increases the hydrostatic pressure at the venular end of the capillary and causes it to become greater than the colloid osmotic pressure thus causing fluid to be forced out of the capillary. If the colloid osmotic pressure becomes low (as when the serum albumin is low in patients with cirrhosis of the liver or in some forms of kidney disease), fluid will be forced out of the capillary.

of fluid circulating in the blood tends to become less. Oedema fluid lying in the subcutaneous and interstitial spaces of the body is then drawn back into the blood stream to help make up for the fluid lost from the blood stream through the kidneys.

Normally there are two forces acting on the fluid which lies in the capillaries. There is the blood pressure in the capillaries which tends to force the fluid through the capillary wall into the interstitial spaces. This force is counteracted by a curious water-holding effect exerted by the albumin molecules in the blood (Fig. 3.5).

In normal people there are usually enough albumin molecules for the water-holding effect to exceed the effect of the blood pressure in forcing fluid out of the capillaries. This means that normally we do not develop oedema.

In congestive cardiac failure, the back-log of blood which the heart has failed to pump away raises the blood pressure in the capillary (tending to force water out) until it exceeds the water-holding effect of the albumin molecules (tending to keep water in). The result is that water is forced out of the capillary and the patient develops oedema.

Patients with liver cirrhosis and the nephrotic syndrome often have low concentrations of albumin in the plasma. The water-holding power of their blood is consequently much reduced because there are fewer molecules of albumin available to hold on to water. These patients also tend to develop oedema.

The oedema found in patients with these three conditions responds well to diuretic therapy.

Nursing observations to be made on patients being treated with diuretics

Close observation of fluid balance on patients receiving diuretic drugs is clearly extremely important. The first reason for this is to ensure that the patients are achieving a good diuretic response. The second is to guard against excessive diuresis as it is possible for patients to pass really enormous amounts of urine soon after being started on a diuretic drug. This is more likely if the patient is very oedematous. The usual means by which fluid intake and output is monitored is by the keeping of a fluid balance chart and this is a fairly time-consuming and quite a difficult task, particularly with a confused or incontinent patient. Regular weighing of the patient is also valuable and reliable and has much to recommend it.

Principles of the management of cardiac failure

The intensity and vigour with which we treat a patient with cardiac failure depends largely on the severity of the condition. In mild cardiac failure, particularly in the elderly, a small dose of a thiazide diuretic used alone is often sufficient. When cardiac failure is more severe, more potent diuretics such as frusemide and bumetanide are required. While the patient's cardiac rhythm remains normal (sinus rhythm) many physicians will attempt to treat their patients with diuretics alone only adding digoxin if the response is poor. Others believe that digoxin is valuable in most cases of cardiac failure and there is still considerable debate on this point. There is no doubt, however, that when a patient is in cardiac failure with uncontrolled atrial fibrillation digitalisation is essential. When cardiac failure presents in its most dramatic form, acute pulmonary oedema due to left ventricular failure, the effect of intravenous frusemide may be dramatic and the introduction of this drug and its successors has revolutionised the treatment of this previously fatal condition. It must not be forgotten that morphine or diamorphine given intravenously are also of great value in left ventricular failure and these drugs are still used in combination with the newer diuretics. Finally, in the most severe and resistant forms of cardiac failure, often the end result of long-standing ischaemic heart disease, valvular heart disease or cardiomyopathy, very large doses of potent diuretics in combination with spironolactone and digoxin are required. As a last desperate measure in these hopeless cases you may occasionally see short-term peritoneal dialysis used in an attempt to remove excessive fluid from the body.

DRUGS USED TO TREAT CARDIAC ARRHYTHMIAS

Introduction

In the last decade many new drugs have become available for the treatment of cardiac arrhythmias. In this field fashions tend to change quickly and no textbook can hope to keep completely up-to-date. The number of agents available is now very large and the contribution in some cases has been rather controversial. This section will cover only these drugs which have some proven value in the prevention or treatment of the arrhythmias.

Digoxin

The actions of digoxin have been fully covered in the last section but as this drug is still frequently used to treat primary rhythm disturbances of the heart it merits further mention. In this context the most common indication for digoxin therapy is atrial fibrillation and the majority of patients with this rhythm abnormality receive the drug. Occasionally old people with relatively slow atrial fibrillation do not require any drug therapy, and sometimes those with atrial fibrillation due to thyrotoxicosis are treated with the beta adrenergic blocking drug propanalol instead. In all other cases of fibrillation whether or not cardiac failure is present, digoxin is still the drug of choice. Other supraventricular rhythm disturbances such as atrial flutter or paroxysmal supraventricular tachycardia may also be treated with digoxin if they fail to respond to other forms of therapy. Again, the presence of cardiac failure may influence the decision to use the drug. Digoxin is of no value in the treatment of ventricular disrhythmias and indeed you should bear in mind that this serious type of rhythm disturbance may be a sign of digoxin toxicity. When digoxin is used to treat arrhythmias the general rules previously laid down about methods of administration, choice of dose and signs and symptoms of toxicity still apply.

Quinidine

Quinidine is derived from the drug quinine which is used to treat malaria. The action of quinidine is in some ways the reverse of digoxin because quinidine decreases the irritability and excitability of heart muscle whereas digoxin increases it. Quinidine is a time honoured remedy which is still widely used because of its efficacy in the treatment of supraventricular and ventricular arrhythmias. For many years quinidine was virtually the only means by which a patient with atrial fibrillation could be converted back into normal sinus rhythm. In general this conversion is only possible in a few patients in whom the arrhythmia has been present for a short time (no longer than 6 weeks). The drug acts by depressing the excitability of the atria and allowing the sino-atrial node to set the pace of cardiac muscle contraction. Nowadays instead of using quinidine to try and convert suitable patients from atrial fibrillation to sinus rhythm, electrical countershock (cardioversion) is used. The ability of quinidine to stabilise excitable myocardial cells makes it a useful drug in the treatment of serious ventricular arrhythmias. It is not usually given in cases of established ventricular tachycardia as it must be given orally and its action is therefore rather slow. These cases are managed by intravenous lignocaine or procainamide (see below) or by electrical cardioversion. Instead, quinidine is reserved for the treatment of ventricular ectopic beats and may to be of value in the abolition of the dangerous variety which occur following a myocardial infarction.

Side effects of quinidine

These are:

1. Idiosyncrasy to quinidine
2. Tinnitus and vertigo with blurring of vision
3. Thrombocytopenia
4. Cardiac failure.

Some patients have idiosyncrasy to quinidine. In these patients the drug causes profound circulatory collapse, that is hypotensive shock. These patients are rare but it is always wise when using quinidine to give a small test dose to your patient. Usually a dose of 120 mg is given. If he feels faint or complains of ringing in the ears (tinnitus) or dizziness (vertigo) or double vision (diplopia) he should not be given the drug.

The low platelet count (thrombocytopenia) which is a rare side effect in patients receiving quinidine, causes bleeding into the skin (purpura) and bleeding from the mucous membranes of the mouth and alimentary tract. When the drug is stopped, the platelet count usually rises promptly.

The ability of quinidine to depress myocardial cells means that in susceptible individuals it may cause cardiac failure to occur and this serious side effect should always be looked for. It may also cause excessive slowing of the heart (bradycardia) and in more serious instances of poisoning cardiac arrest can occur.

Dosage of quinidine

This varies from patient to patient but an average dose is 300 mg four to six times a day. Nowadays a slow release preparation is available which only has to be given twice daily.

Procainamide

This drug has a similar action to quinidine in that it is a powerful depressant of the excitability of heart muscle. Its main uses are the rapid control of ventricular tachycardia and the treatment and prevention of ventricular ectopic beats following myocardial infarction. Procainamide may also be of value in the management of certain supraventricular arrhythmias and is effective in the treatment of atrial tachycardia which is sometimes a side effect of digoxin therapy. In the emergency situation it is always given intravenously, usually a bolus injection followed by a continuous infusion but it can be given orally thereafter for the prevention of further arrhythmias. The problems associated with the rapid elimination of procainamide from the body and the necessity for frequent oral administration can be avoided by the use of a special formulation which slowly releases the drug into the intestine and thence into the blood stream, providing a fairly steady concentration of the drug over a fairly long period of time, and obviating the need for very frequent dosing. Procainamide is a dangerous and a difficult drug to use and its correct use calls for skill on the doctor's part. You will not be called upon to administer this drug yourself but you may be called upon to assist when it is being given. Procainamide is administered *slowly* intravenously. The two dangers associated with its use are cardiac standstill and extreme hypotension. The onset of cardiac standstill is sudden and for this reason when the drug is given, electrocardiographic control is necessary. The doctor monitors the heart rate and rhythm on the electrocardiogram. As soon as he sees that the ventricular tachycardia has reverted to sinus rhythm, he stops the injection.

You may have to watch for the second complication of procainamide therapy, extreme hypotension, by constantly taking the blood pressure (at intervals of one minute or thereabouts). If the systolic blood pressure falls below 100 mm of mercury this is a warning to stop the injection or to continue with extreme caution.

Lignocaine

Originally this agent was used as a local anaesthetic but it has been discovered to be of value in the treatment of cardiac arrhythmias by virtue of its action in lowering the excitability of the heart muscle. The advantage of lignocaine over procainamide is that the force of contraction of the heart muscle does not appear to be decreased to the same extent. This drug is of the greatest value in suppressing arrythmias arising in the ventricles such as ventricular ectopic beats or ventricular tachycardia, a condition which is particularly dangerous in that it is associated with a very poor cardiac output and may precede the development of ventricular fibrillation. In this condition the ventricular wall shimmers without effectively ejecting any blood into the peripheral circulation. Unless treated, death ensues within a matter of minutes.

The myocardium is very liable to ventricular arrhythmias after a myocardial infarction and if you work in a coronary care unit it is likely that you will see lignocaine being used fairly frequently. The drug can be injected intravenously without the necessity for ECG monitoring which exists with procainamide. A typical dose might be 5 ml of a 2 per cent solution (equivalent to 100 mg). If it is necessary to set up a continuous intravenous infusion of lignocaine, ECG control becomes mandatory, however, because in these circumstances the drug may accumulate in the blood and cause disturbance of conduction in the heart.

Some patients become very agitated and tremulous when given intravenous lignocaine; confusion and convulsions may occur and the drug may also cause increased sweating. Some patients experience a feeling of impending doom during lignocaine injections which is particularly terrifying for them. Lignocaine is inactivated by the liver and individuals whose livers are badly congested due to cardiac failure will break down the drug rather slowly; this means that these patients are at greater risk of developing toxicity during therapy and they may require a reduction in the dosage of lignocaine given to them.

Disopyramide

This is a relatively new drug which has a quinidine-like action and appears effective in the treatment and prevention of supraventricular and ventricular arrhythmias. It is probably less toxic than quinidine but may induce cardiac failure in susceptible individuals. It is usually administered by the oral route.

Atropine

This drug is also covered in the section in gastrointestinal drugs and you may find its inclusion here suprising. In fact because of its sympathetic-like effect and its ability to speed up the heart it is of great value in the treatment of bradycardia. Excessive slowing of the heart is a common complication in myocardial infarction and early treatment with atropine given intravenously will often restore the rate and also improve the cardiac output and blood pressure. Occasionally if the patient is treated quickly atropine may reverse the dangerous condition known as heartblock, although this complication usually requires insertion into the heart of a temporary pacemaker wire. The most common side effect of atropine is drying of the mouth due to inhibition of the salivary glands but excessive quickening of the heart and even supraventricular tachycardia may follow large doses. Occasionally atropine will induce acute glaucoma in the elderly.

Isoprenaline

Complete heart block is a condition in which none of the atrial contractions are transmitted down the bundle of His to the ventricles. When this happens the ventricles beat at their own pace of about 30–40 heats per minute (idioventricular rhythm). This is a serious situation because the ventricles may not eject enough blood at these rates to keep the patient conscious. Heart block occuring after myocardial infarction may be associated with rates even less than 30 per minute and death may be imminent. The correct procedure in these instances is to insert a device known as a transvenous pacing catheter into the heart starting the insertion from a peripheral vein in the forearm or the internal jugular vein in the neck.

If this device is not available it may be possible to increase the ventricular rate by the administration of isoprenaline. This is a very specialised technique which requires an initial testing of the patient's response to the drug which in these cases is usually given intravenously. The danger is of the precipitation by isoprenaline of ventricular arrhythmias. For this reason the patient is monitored by ECG during administration of the drug and at the first sign of ventricular ectopic beats or ventricular tachycardia therapy is stopped.

The technique of administration is to add 2 ml of a solution of isoprenaline (containing 2 mg of drug) to 500 ml normal saline or dextrose and to deliver the infusion initially at the rate of 20 drops per minute. The doctor will adjust the flow depending on the response of the patient.

Beta adrenergic blocking drugs

The sympathetic nervous system sends fibres to, among other

areas, the heart, the lungs and arterioles in muscle. These cardiac, pulmonary and arteriolar fibres are known as beta adrenergic nerves and they are different from sympathetic branches in other areas such as arterioles in skin, (alpha adrenergic) because some drugs can block transmission of nervous impulses at beta adrenergic endings but not at alpha endings; conversely, there are agents which block transmission of alpha adrenergic impulses but not beta ones. Thus the sympathetic nervous system can be considered as being divided into at least two parts (alpha and beta) which can be distinguished from each other in how they respond to alpha and beta blocking drugs. Beta adrenergic stimulation increases both the pulse rate and the amount of work done by the heart. It follows that drugs which block this stimulation (beta blocking drugs) might be expected to cause a slowing of the pulse rate and a decrease in the work of the heart. This is indeed what happens in practice when these drugs are given to patients.

Uses of beta blocking drugs

There are three main areas where beta blockings drugs are effective:

1. Treatment of cardiac arrhythmias
2. Treatment of angina pectoris (pp. 61–62).
3. Treatment of hypertension (pp. 71–72).

Cardiac arrhythmias particularly liable to respond to beta blocking drugs are those occurring in the thyrotoxic patient (atrial fibrillation), or those occurring as a result of digoxin toxicity. Paroxysmal supraventricular tachycardia, a condition characterised by the abrupt onset of paroxysms of very fast regular atrial contractions, also may respond to these drugs and in this situation they offer an alternative to the use of digoxin. Beta blocking agents produce their desired effects by protecting the irritable heart, that is the heart which is likely to develop a tachycardia, from unwanted sympathetic stimulation.

Similar considerations underlie the usefulness of these agents in the treatment of angina pectoris. Essentially angina occurs when the heart muscle works sufficiently hard or fast so as to outstrip its blood supply. Sympathetic stimulation drives the heart to work more rapidly and with increased force of contraction and when this stimulation is blocked the effect is a decrease in cardiac work.

We all of us are subject to cardiac adrenergic stimulation in our daily lives. For example, it has been shown that people who have to stand up and speak in public in front of others (e.g. nurses in a tutorial group or answering questions from the tutor) attain heart rates of the order of 160 to 200 beats per minute. Car drivers often reach similar rates during ordinary motoring through routine traffic conditions. Beta adrenergic blocking drugs are thus particularly useful for the angina patient because they prevent the development of cardiac responses like those discussed above and thus prevent to a very large extent the development of attacks of angina pectoris. Indeed these agents may be regarded as having a long-lasting action in angina and they thus contrast very favourably with glyceryl trinitrate which has a short lived action.

Many patients with hypertension can now be controlled satisfactorily with beta blocking drugs. In hypertension the heart pumps blood into the circulation with an increased force and this is one of the factors responsible for the increase in blood pressure. When the sympathetic drive to the heart is blocked by treatment the force of cardiac contraction is considerably reduced and one effect of this is to be seen in the lowering of the blood pressure witout the unpleasant and potentially dangerous complication of postural hypotension which occurs with some of the older drugs.

In practice it takes about 2 to 6 weeks before the correct dose of beta blocking drug is found for the individual patient and during this time the dose of drug is built up from an initially small one to the correct one needed to maintain the diastolic pressure, at 90 mm Hg or less.

Side effects

To a very large extent it is unfair to describe the complications of treatment with beta blocking drugs as *side effects,* since a knowledge of the mode of action of the agents and a little reflection would allow you to *predict* what additional effects might result during beta blockade. Therefore the term 'side effects' might be better replaced by the term 'unwanted actions'. These considerations hold good for very many drugs, but particularly so for beta blockers.

Sympathetic beta stimulation in the lungs causes dilation of the bronchioles and smaller bronchi. Accordingly *bronchoconstriction* might be expected to accompany blockade of beta stimulation and this is indeed the case. In patients with normal lungs this is of little consequence but in those with bronchial asthma the use of beta blockers is contraindicated because an intractable attack of asthma may be induced. You should always ask your patient if he has ever had asthma or lung trouble in childhood before giving him a beta blocking drug for the first time.

Cardiac failure, particularly *left ventricular failure* may be precipitated during treatment with these agents and is particularly likely to occur within the first ten days. If the myocardium is having to work hard to prevent the patient from going into cardiac failure the addition of a beta blocking agent which *reduces* the amount of work done by the cardiac muscle may tip the balance against the near-failing heart and frank cardiac failure may ensue.

The list of beta blocking drugs available for use is now long and rather confusing. Propranolol was the first drug to be widely used, followed by practolol and oxyprenolol. Newer additions include metroprolol, atenolol, pindolol and a number of others. The differences between these drugs are not very great and we will confine our discussion to the first three agents.

Propranolol (Inderal)

This agent is effective in the treatment of certain arrhythmias. It is usually given orally three or four times a day but in emergency situations, for example, in the treatment of digoxin toxicity, it can be given intravenously in small doses (of the order of 0.5 to 1.0 mg). The total intravenous dose should never exceed 5 mg and if doses up to this magnitude are required the drug is injected very slowly over a period of 10 to 15 minutes.

Apart from precipitating asthmatic attacks or cardiac failure, propranolol may also cause drowsiness in a few individuals. Some patients find that they have to discontinue therapy because of very vivid dreams or nightmares. These latter side effects suggest that the drug may have an action on the brain. Occasionally skin rashes occur.

Oxprenolol (Trasicor)

An advantage of this drug is that it is less likely than propranolol to induce attacks of asthma in susceptible individuals; in addition it is less likely to cause heart failure. The indications for its use are the same as for propanolol.

Practolol

Practolol shares with oxyprenolol a degree of cardio selectivity in that it is less likely to produce asthma. Use of this drug is now confined to intravenous administration for the emergency treatment of supraventricular arrhythmias. The reason for this restriction is that some patients on long term treatment with practolol were found to have developed chronic skin rashes and inflammation of the eye, middle ear and peritoneum. These serious complications led to fears about safety of the other beta blocking drugs but so far none of the other members of this group has definitely been associated with the so-called 'oculo-muco-cutaneous syndrome'. The oral form of practolol is now no longer available.

Nursing observations on patients being treated with beta blocking drugs

1. You should look for attacks of wheezing which might suggest the beginning of an asthmatic attack. Therapy must be stopped at once pending further examination of the patient by the doctor.
2. Signs of breathlessness or swelling of the ankles suggest the development of cardiac failure and again constitute a clear reason for withdrawing the beta blocker.
3. Skin rashes in patients receiving practolol raise the possibility of the development of systemic lupus erythematosus. The drug must be stopped until further investigations have been done.

Principles of the management of cardiac arrhythmias

The wide range of drugs now used for the treatment of various cardiac arrhythmias is very confusing and in this field there is considerable debate as to which drug is the best in different situations. It is not possible for this book to cover all the available agents and discussion has to be confined to those in common use.

In general, established atrial fibrillation is treated with digoxin although some exceptions are noted in the section on digoxin in cardiac arrhythmias. Paroxysmal supraventricular tachycardia is generally treated with an intravenous beta blocking drug, usually practolol or propranolol, with continuation of oral propranolol to prevent recurrence. Resistant cases of supraventricular tachycardia may be treated by electrical cardioversion or by digitalisation, particularly when cardiac failure is present. Ventricular arrhythmias are particularly dangerous as they may be a forerunner of ventricular fibrillation, which is inevitably fatal if not treated immediately by high voltage countershock. Prevention of ventricular arrhythmias is understandably our main concern, particularly following myocardial infarction. Intravenous lignocaine, usually by continuous infusion, is most commonly used in the acute situation although procainamide may occasionally be more effective. Lignocaine cannot be given orally so preventive therapy is continued with the oral form of procainamide, quinidine or disopyramide. All the drugs used in the treatment of arrhythmias have potentially serious side effects and patients receiving them are usually nursed initially in an intensive care area with continuous monitoring. They may, however, continued therapy in a general ward and the nursing staff must be alert to the possibility of development of unwanted effects such as bradycardia, cardiac failure or bronchospasm.

DRUGS USED TO TREAT ANGINA PECTORIS

Glyceryl trinitrate and the beta blocking drugs are the agents of most value in the treatment of patients with angina pectoris.

Factors contributing to cardiac pain

The heart is a very active muscular organ. On account of its activity the heart muscle produces a great deal of energy. A byproduct of this energy is the formation of many metabolites, e.g. lactic acid. These metabolites result from the breakdown of energy-giving substances in the heart muscle. They are metabolised by the oxygen carried in the arterial blood via the branches of the coronary arteries. It often happens that due to atheroma, the lumen of some of the coronary arteries becomes much reduced and in some instances may be completely blocked. The result of this is a decreased amount of blood reaching some parts of the cardiac muscle. Accordingly, the metabolites within these areas are not broken down and their concentration increases in the tissues. The patient experiences pain when the level of these metabolites becomes too high and this pain is called angina pectoris.

Glyceryl trinitrate

The action of glyceryl trinitrate is to cause intense vasodilatation of the arteries all over the body, including the *normal* coronary arteries, The intense vasodilatation causes a fall in the peripheral resistance (see p. 63 for further explanation of this effect). When resistance falls, the heart has to pump against less pressure and therefore the amount of cardiac work is lowered. This in turn requires the consumption of less oxygen by the myocardial cells bringing the needs of the heart muscle closer to the capacity of the narrowed arteries to supply blood to the heart. This effect produces rapid relief of the attack of angina. Vasodilatation of *diseased* coronary arteries probably is not possible as these structures are rendered rigid with calcified plaques of atheroma.

Method of administration of glyceryl trinitrate

You must instruct your patient to hold a crushed tablet of glyceryl trinitrate under his tongue until it has dissolved because this drug is absorbed through the buccal mucosa. Each tablet of glyceryl trinitrate contains 0.5 mg of the drug.

Many patients typically experience angina pectoris on exercise or during effort. It is sometimes possible for patients to prevent an attack of angina by taking a tablet just before performing an action which they know brings on an attack. For example, one patient who had to climb 12 steps to get to his work every morning usually developed angina pectoris on the seventh or eighth stair. This always caused him to stop until the attack wore off and he used to feel very embarrassed about stopping while people stared at him. This man found that if he took a tablet of glyceryl trinitrate a minute or so before he came to the steps, he was able to climb them with relative ease.

In general if an attack of angina has not cleared after two tablets then it is unlikely to respond to further treatment. However, patients with many attacks of angina may consume 20 or more tablets in one day and as glyceryl trinitrate is short acting and its side effects are not serious this does not constitute a risk and they should not be discouraged from this habit.

Side effects of glyceryl trinitrate

The side effects of this drug are directly related to its action in causing vasodilatation. Skin flushing occurs, sometimes to a remarkable extent, in susceptible individuals. Some patients feel slightly dizzy after taking the drug and occasionally elderly patients may faint. A more inconvenient side effect is throbbing headache. The intracerebral arteries are painful when dilated because the walls of these arteries carry pain-sensitive nerve endings which are stimulated when the vessel wall expands. Each pulse beat distends these arteries a little bit more and the headache throbs with each pulse beat.

Long acting nitrates

Over the years a number of nitrate drugs have been produced which are swallowed rather than placed under the tongue. The principle behind this is that absorption from the gut will be slower and therefore more prolonged relief of angina will follow. In practice this treatment has been disappointing and at present there is no real evidence that these drugs have any beneficial effect in angina.

Beta blocking drugs in angina

A large number of drugs in this group has already been mentioned in the section on cardiac arrhythmias. Beta blockers may be very effective in reducing the number of attacks of angina in any one day but are of no value in the acute attack, when only glyceryl trinitrate is effective. Patients are usually started on a fairly small dose of these drugs, for instance propranolol 10 or 20 mg four times daily, and this is gradually increased until the symptoms improve or the resting heart rate falls to 60 beats per minute or below. Beta blocking drugs lower both the heart rate and the cardiac output and therefore reduce the amount of work the heart has to do. Another consideration is that the patient who anticipates an attack of angina on say walking up a hill or a flight of stairs will experience a rise in heart rate prior to exerting himself due to an increase in nervous impulses to the heart. This anticipation of difficulty will hasten the onset of angina. Beta blocking drugs block this nervous effect and therefore delay or even abolish the subsequent attack of pain. As in other situations beta blocking drugs may induce cardiac failure or bronchospasm in susceptible individuals. Patients receiving these drugs for angina must be closely observed for these unwanted effects.

Principles of the management of angina

Many patients with relatively mild angina, particularly the elderly, can be managed with glyceryl trinitrate alone. When attacks of pain are more frequent and severe and start interfering with the patient's life, then they are usually started on a beta blocking drug and this therapy may prove very effective indeed. Many patients with mild or moderate angina survive for twenty years or more with virtually no therapy. Nowadays younger patients with severe crippling angina are sometimes considered for surgery at an early stage, particularly if they have failed to respond to beta blocking drugs. The operation uses a vein graft to by-pass occluded segments of coronary arteries and this may dramatically relieve the most severe cases of angina. It should be remembered that no treatment currently available for angina has been shown to definitely prevent subsequent myocardial infarction or to prolong life.

DRUGS USED TO TREAT PATIENTS WITH HYPERTENSION

Any discussion of drugs in this class (sometimes called antihypertensive drugs or agents) must necessarily be preceded by a brief recapitulation of the physiology of the factors responsible for control of the blood pressure. An understanding of these factors is essential for a clear grasp not only of the actions of antihypertensive agents but also of their side effects.

Factors controlling the blood pressure

There are three factors which control the normal blood pressure in man. These are:

1. The viscosity of the blood
2. The cardiac output
3. The peripheral resistance.

The viscosity of the blood is probably not very important for it is not changed in diseases where the blood pressure changes nor is it changed by anti-hypertensive drugs.

The cardiac output is determined principally by the venous return of blood to the heart, by the heart rate and by the amount of sympathetic nerve stimulation delivered to the myocardial cells. The greater the sympathetic stimulation, the greater the cardiac work and the higher the blood pressure. You will recall from you knowledge of physiology that the more blood in the ventricles the greater the force of heart muscle contraction (and therefore the greater the pressure of the blood ejected from the heart). The less the blood in the heart the less the force of heart muscle contraction and the lower the blood pressure (Starling's law). Those of you who have soaked for too long in a hot bath may have noticed that when you stand up after your bath you suddenly feel faint for a second or two. This is because the heat of the water has dilated your arterioles and capillaries and the blood has pooled there. When you stand up gravity prevents the blood in the dilated arterioles from returning immediately to your heart through the venules. This sudden fall in venous return to the heart causes a sharp drop in blood pressure, as predicted from Starling's law, and you feel faint for a few moments until matters right themselves (by arteriolar vasoconstriction).

The peripheral resistance is a major factor in determining blood pressure. It is principally the calibre of the lumen of the arterioles which control the peripheral resistance. The lumen of the arteriole changes in diameter depending whether the smooth muscle in its wall is constricted or relaxed. The state of contraction or relaxation of the arteriolar wall musculature is under the control of a centre in the brain (the vasomotor centre). This centre exerts its influence on the arterioles via the autonomic nervous system the activity of which cannot in most of us be voluntarily regulated.

You will recall that the autonomic nervous system has two kinds of nerve fibres, sympathetic and parasympathetic. This is illustrated in Figure 3.6. The nerve fibres of the parasympathetic system transmit their electrical impulses through their ganglia by releasing the chemical substance acetylcholine. These fibres also stimulate the target organ by releasing acetylcholine. The sympathetic system on the other hand transmits acetylcholine at its ganglia but stimulates its target organ by releasing noradrenaline.

The sympathetic system can be shown to be composed of at least two parts, the so called alpha and beta adrenergic fibres. This distinction is made because it has been discovered that some drugs block transmission of nerve impulses only at some (beta) sympathetic nerve endings (for example in heart muscle, bronchioles and arterioles in muscle) whereas others act on different (alpha) sympathetic endings (for example in peripheral arterioles in skin and in the viscera) leaving heart muscle and bronchioles unaffected.

It follows therefore that a drug which blocks the release of acetylcholine will interfere with the activity of both the parasympathetic and the sympathetic nerve fibres and will produce side effects related to disturbances of both these systems. A drug which blocks the release of noradrenaline will interfere only with the sympathetic nerve fibres and will produce side effects related only to the sympathetic nervous system. Finally, a drug which *selectively* blocks beta sympathetic nerve endings will selectively lower the work done by the heart and most unwanted effects of generalised sympathetic blockade will be absent.

The parasympathetic fibres do not innervate arterioles, the only autonomic control of these being by the sympathetic fibres which cause arteriolar vasoconstriction and therefore a rise in blood pressure. Accordingly when the effect of these fibres are removed, either by ganglion-blocking drugs or by adrenergic-blocking agents the arterioles dilate causing a fall in blood pressure with decrease in the peripheral resistance.

Notice that a fall in the peripheral resistance means pooling of blood in the periphery with less venous return to the heart. This means a further drop in blood pressure and, as you might expect from the example quoted on the physiology of the hot bath, the maximum fall in blood pressure occurs when the patient stands erect. This is called postural hypotension.

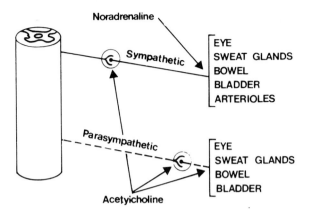

Fig. 3.6. The sympathetic and parasympathetic nerve fibres. Ganglion-blocking drugs act at the sites of release of acetylcholine and thus block both nerve fibres. Adrenergic-blocking drugs act at the site of release of noradrenaline and block the action of the sympathetic nerve fibres.

There is no single ideal drug available for the treatment of hypertension. A vast number of drugs have been used in the past. This chapter describes those that are still in general use. It does not mention drugs that were once used but are now fast becoming obsolete nor does it mention current drugs on trial in clinical practice but awaiting final assessment.

GANGLION-BLOCKING DRUGS

The term ganglion-blocking drug means that the substance in question blocks the release of acetylcholine in both the parasympathetic and sympathetic autonomic ganglia. All of the drugs in this group tend to have the same side effects because of this action and differences between them relate only to methods of administration or reliability of absorption from the alimentary tract.

Side effects of the ganglion-blocking drugs

The autonomic nervous system innervates the salivary glands, the ciliary muscle of the eye, the sweat glands, the smooth muscle of arteriolar walls, the smooth muscles and sphincters of the bowel and bladder and in the male of the muscles of the corpora cavernosa. It is not difficult to understand that blocking the action of the autonomic nervous system besides causing a fall in blood pressure will give rise to the following side effects.

1. Impairment in the power of accommodation of the eye. This is due to interference with the function of the ciliary muscle and is experienced by the patient as blurring of vision.

2. Reduction in sweating and dryness of the mouth. A constantly dry mouth can be a most unpleasant experience.

3. Constipation and difficulty with micturition. These two side effects may be especially severe in elderly patients who may be costive and have a tendency to difficulty with micturition (in men because of prostate enlargement).

4. Impotence. The failure to sustain an erection may be extremely worrying to youger patients and many of them ask to have ganglion-blocking drugs discontinued because of this side effect.

5. Postural hypotension. The reasons for this have already been discussed. The condition may occur quite dramatically. Your patient receiving treatment with a ganglion-blocking drug could swing his legs over the edge of his bed, try to stand on the floor, become unconscious and collapse due to extreme hypotension. As soon as he is lying on the floor he will regain consciousness because his cerebral circulation returns rapidly.

Although at one time they were the only effective drugs available, ganglion-blocking agents have been virtually completely replaced by modern drugs with more selective action which do not produce the long list of troublesome side effects noted above.

Pentolinium (Ansolysen)

Pentolinium is really the only ganglion-blocker still in use. It is valuable in the emergency treatment of severe hypertension when a subcutaneous injection of 1 or 2 mg will produce a sharp fall in blood pressure within 10 minutes. To some extent the fall in blood pressure is dependent on the patient's posture and the drug's effect can be greatly enhanced if the patient is placed semi-upright. Equally the effects of the drug can be partly reversed and the blood pressure elevated by raising the food of the bed. These changes are a reflection of the extent of 'pooling' of the blood in the legs which occurs when the autonomic ganglia are blocked by this drug.

ADRENERGIC-BLOCKING DRUGS

Adrenergic-blocking drugs selectively block the transmission of the nerve impulses in the sympathetic nervous system. They do this by blocking the release of noradrenaline from the sympathetic nerve fibres at the level of their target organ. Because they do not block the parasympathetic nerve fibres the side effects with these drugs are very much less than the side effects of the ganglion-blocking agents. Dryness of the mouth, difficulties with micturition, impotence and blurring of vision are less commonly observed than with ganglion-blockers, but in men failure of ejaculation frequently occurs. The best known of this group of drugs are guanethidine, bethanidine and debrisoquine. All adrenergic-blocking drugs have their hypotensive action antagonised by amphetamine, ephedrine and the tricyclic anti-depressant drugs such as imipramine. If you hypertensive patient requires treatment for depression it may be necessary for him to have his anti-hypertensive therapy changed.

Guanethidine

This drug has a slow onset of action and the effects of a single dose may last for as long as a week or more. Two things follow from this. Firstly, your patient requires to take only one daily dose. This is usually given in the morning. Secondly, it is wise to allow almost a week to elapse before increasing the dose. This is because the long action of the drug produces a cumulative effect where some of last week's dose may be having an effect next week. Accordingly if patients are brought into hospital and are started on guanethidine it may take some time before a dose is reached which is suitable to control that particular patient. It is usual to start a patient on 10 mg a day and to increase this by 10 mg per day every sixth or seventh day depending on his blood pressure response. You may notice that patients who showed good and fairly steady control of their blood pressure in hospital often have slightly higher blood pressure readings on their return to the clinic for surveillance. One simple remedy which is often quite effective at this point in bringing the blood pressure down to an acceptable level is to add a thiazide diuretic such as chlorothiazide or bendrofluazide to their regimen of treatment. The midly hypotensive effect of these agents in conjunction with guanethidine often stabilises the blood pressure.

Side effects of guanethidine

The side effects of this drug are much milder than those of the ganglion-blocking agents. Diarrhoea occurs in some patients. This is due to the unopposed action of the parasympathetic nervous system producing hypermotility of the bowel and relax-ation of its smooth muscle sphincters once the normal opposing effect of the sympathetic nervous system has been removed by guanethidine. The diarrhoea usually clears up spontaneously.

Nasal stuffiness is experienced by a few patients but is not troublesome. A curious and so far unexplained finding is that some patients receiving this drug develop pitting ankle oedema. In the majority of cases this is mild but in a few it is marked. The swelling usually responds to diuretic therapy.

Postural hypotension is most troublesome in the morning especially on first rising from bed. You should warn your patient about this.

Bethanidine

Bethanidine is a fairly potent hypotensive agent with a much faster onset and shorter duration of action than guanethidine. Postural hypotension can be a serious problem with this drug. As older patients are more at risk from cerebral damage as a result of a sudden fall in blood pressure this drug tends to be reserved for the younger patient with severe hypertension.

Although it has to be taken twice or thrice daily in contrast to the single daily dose of guanethidine, bethanidine has the advantage that it does not cause diarrhoea. A typical dose initially is 5 mg twice daily increasing gradually to 30 mg thrice daily if the lower dose is not effective.

Debrisoquine (Declinax)

Like bethanidine this adrenergic blocking-agent does not cause diarrhoea. It too has a shorter duration of action than guanethidine and has to be taken two to three times a day.

A typical starting dose is 10 mg twice daily increasing to a maximum of 40 mg thrice daily. As with the older adrenergic blocking drugs, postural hypotension may occur.

Nursing observations on patients receiving treatment with ganglion-blocking or adrenergic-blocking agents

1. One nursing observation which it is important to make when a patient is being treated with these drugs is to record the blood pressure not only when the patient is lying in bed but also when he is standing. In normal individuals the systolic and diastolic blood pressures are slightly (about 10 mm of mercury) lower when standing than when lying down. In patients on any kind of treatment with hypotensive drugs this normal phenomenon may be slightly exaggerated and differences of 20 or even 30 mm of mercury may be observed in the blood pressure between lying and standing. Differences greater than this indicate that your patient is liable to develop clinically obvious effects such as fainting from his postural hypotension. It is important to know about this and to take action to prevent it. You will be able to imagine many situations in everyday life where it might be extremely dangerous or even fatal to lose consciousness (for example crossing the street).

2. If your patient complains of a dry mouth or of blurring of vision, this should be reported to sister. It is wise to check that he is not experiencing undue difficulty with defaecation or micturition. This is especially so in elderly patients in whom acute retention of urine may develop very suddenly.

Methyldopa (Aldomet)

The mode of action of methyldopa appears to be that it is converted in the body to a derivative of noradrenaline. This derivative then blocks the effect of true noradrenaline on the peripheral arterioles thereby causing vasodilatation and a fall in blood pressure. Methyldopa causes less postural hypotension than guanethidine, bethanidine or debrisoquine.

Methyldopa is a very useful anti-hypertensive agent and is much more widely used nowadays than the other drugs mentioned above. It has an action of moderate intensity in controlling the blood pressure and is especially useful in treating patients with hypertension secondary to some diseases of the kidney. It is given orally and is well absorbed. A typical daily dose of this drug might be 250 mg taken four times a day.

Side effects of methyldopa

Side effects are usually mild. An interesting observation which you will be able to confirm quite readily for yourself is that patients given the drug often develop marked drowsiness during the first few days of treatment. The cause of this is unknown and it usually clears up spontaneously Occasionally methyldopa causes a haemolytic anaemia. It appears that in a few individuals the drug causes the body to form antibodies to the red corpuscles which are then destroyed and removed from the circulation. This will result in anaemia and jaundice resulting from the ecessive breakdown of haemoglobin.

Methyldopa should not be given to patients with a history of liver disease because rarely the drug may cause a form of hepatitis (inflammation of the liver).

Clonidine

Clonidine is a moderately effective anti-hypertensive drug which appears to act both centrally on the sympathetic control centre in the brain and peripherally on the arterioles; the net effect is to cause a mild vasodilatation with lowering of blood pressure.

The drug is used in very small doses, for example an initial dose of 0.1 mg thrice daily is usual. Paradoxically if very large doses are used the blood pressure may actually increase and this may be because the structure of the drug is rather similar to the structure of the sympathetic amines in the body and in high concentrations it has a similar action to these substances.

Side effects include oedema due to retention of fluid by the body, constipation and dryness of the mouth. Some patients become depressed during treatment and then the drug must be stopped. Others develop extreme drowsiness and have to stop clonidine. Clonidine should not be stopped suddenly as this may occasionally precipitate a severe hypertensive crisis. Withdrawal of the drug should be gradual.

Reserpine

Reserpine has been in use for many years. It acts by depleting noradrenaline at the post-ganglionic nerve endings of the sympathetic nervous system. It also act centrally, depressing the activity of sympathetic centres in the brain. This reduces the degree of vasoconstriction of the arterioles and lowers the blood pressure. It is a mild anti-hypertensive agent and is often used in combination with other drugs. It is more popular in the United States and Continent of Europe than it is in the United Kingdom.

Side effects of reserpine

For a drug which has only a mild action which benefits the patient only slightly, reserpine has some common side effects. The most serious of these is its tendency to produce severe mental depression. Patients who become depressed while receiving reserpine may contemplate and even commit suicide. This depressive illness may persist even when reserpine is discontinued. The greater the dose the more likely is this complication of treatment. The drug can also cause a syndrome which resembles Parkinson's Disease with marked tremor and rigidity of the muscles.

BETA BLOCKING DRUGS IN HYPERTENSION

Some of the actions of these agents have already been discussed in the sections on cardiac arrhythmias and angina pectoris. In the recent past this group of drugs has become very widely used in the management of hypertension and they are probably the treatment of choice either alone or in combination with other agents in high blood pressure of mild or moderate severity. Most experience has been gained with propranolol and this is still the most widely used beta blocking drug. In general, the doses required in hypertension are higher than those used in angina or arrhythmias. Typical doses of propranolol in hypertension vary between 200 and 600 mg per day. A slow release preparation of another member of this group, oxyprenolol, is now available and some of the newer drugs, for instance atenolol, may be given as a single dose each day. This has the advantage of simplicity and is thought to improve the patient's compliance with drug therapy.

The side effects of beta blockers have already been discussed in detail but in general they tend to be less common and much less severe than those which accompany use of ganglion blockers or adrenergic blocking agents such as guanethidine or methyldopa. This group of drugs therefore is valuable for treatment of hypertension in all age groups.

VASODILATOR DRUGS

A number of drugs have the property of lowering blood pressure by causing dilatation of the arterioles. They do this by a direct action on the smooth muscle in the vessel wall.

Diazoxide

A derivative of the thiadiazine group of diuretics, diazoxide, has been found to possess the property of acutely lowering the blood pressure after intravenous injection. It is therefore of value in hypertensive encephalopathy and in eclamptic toxaemia of pregnancy. Diazoxide is a potent vasodilator and acts directly on the smooth muscle in the arteriolar walls. An interesting and important point is that the injection must be rapid as diazoxide binds to serum proteins in the circulation as well as smooth muscle cells. During a slow intravenous injection the drug is 'mopped up' in the circulation and very little is left free to produce the desired effect. Diazoxide is now a very popular drug for the rapid lowering of blood pressure in severe hypertension. The dose given tends to lie between 100 and 300 mg. In general the patient should initially be given a small amount to assess the effect, as large doses such as 300 mg will sometimes produce catastrophic hypotension. The drug has a relatively short duration of action and injections may have to be repeated several times over 24 hours while a more long-acting agent is introduced. Diazoxide cannot be given as long term therapy as it inhibits the release of insulin from the pancreas and so induces diabetes.

Hydrallazine

This is a potent vasodilator drug which has been in use for many years and has recently come back into fashion. It is frequently given intramuscularly in acute hypertensive crisis but unlike diazoxide is suitable for long-term oral therapy. It is thought to be particularly valuable in the management of hypertension associated with renal disease as it does seem to depress renal function to the same extent as some other drugs. In long-term therapy it is frequently used in combination with other drugs. Side effects include palpitations, flushing and tachycardia. In chronic use hydrallazine is renowned for its propensity to induce the rare disease, systemic lupus erythematosus. Side effects are thought to be much less common if the total daily dose is kept below 200 mg.

Prazosin

This is a relatively new drug which like diazoxide and hydrallazine lowers blood pressure by a selective action on arteriolar smooth muscle. It is only available in the oral form and therefore is not normally used in hypertensive crisis. Used alone or in combination with other drugs it is useful in the long-term management of hypertension. During long-term therapy side effects are not common but shortly after introduction of the drug it was noticed that patients occasionally developed severe hypotension and became unconscious after the very first dose. To avoid this alarming side effect, patients should always be given a very small dose (usually 0.5 mg) to assess the effect before commenced on regular therapy.

Principles of the management of hypertension

It is impossible to lay down hard and fast rules about the management of hypertension as this tends to be a matter of personal preference and, as in the management of the arrhythmias, fashion changes quickly following the introduction of new drugs. In general, mild hypertension with a diastolic blood pressure of less than 110 mm with no associated effects such as left ventricular hypertrophy or renal damage is usually treated with a single drug such as a thiazide diuretic or a beta blocking agent. Moderate hypertension, diastolic blood pressure 110 to 130 mm, may require two drugs, say a beta blocking agent or methyldopa in conjunction with a thiazide diuretic. Severe hypertension with left ventricular hypertrophy, renal and retinal damage usually require two or even three drugs used in combination. In this situation some of the older and very potent drugs such as bethanidine may be required, but as stated above side effects are commoner with these agents. There is no ideal remedy and in an individual patient large doses of a number of drugs may be tried before ideal control of the blood pressure is achieved. At present a combination of a beta blocking agent, a diuretic and a vasodilating agent such as hydrallazine is popular for the management of severe hypertension. It is important to remember that blood pressure rises with increasing age and the elderly frequently have blood pressure readings that would be considered very abnormal in younger patients. For this reason hypertension is not usually treated in the over 70s unless it is exceptionally severe. In this age group the results of treatment, for instance postural hypotension, may be more of a risk than not treating the patient at all.

DRUGS USED TO TREAT PATIENTS WITH SHOCK

Acute hypotension can arise from a number of causes. The severer causes, and those which demand treatment are associated with the clinical picture of circulatory inadequacy (shock) and include such conditions as myocardial infarction, septicaemia, trauma and haemorrhage. The drugs once used to elevate the blood pressure non-specifically in these conditions worked by mimicking the action of the sympathetic nervous system on the smooth muscle wall of the arterioles. They caused contraction of this wall thus producing intense vasoconstriction, increased peripheral resistance and a consequent sharp rise in blood pressure.

The danger of vasoconstrictors is that they raised blood pressure at the expense of perfusion of vital organs such as the kidney and may have helped to bring about complications such as anuria. For this reason these agents are no longer used in the treatment of the various types of shock.

If low blood pressure results from loss of blood the correct approach is to replace blood. If shock is due to poor cardiac output following myocardial infarction, digoxin may be required. Septicaemic shock requires vigorous use of appropriate antibiotics.

DRUGS USED TO TREAT PATIENTS WITH DISORDERS OF THE PERIPHERAL CIRCULATION

One would like in some diseases to cause vasodilatation of the arterioles in the skin of the extremities. For example, in peripheral vascular disease the skin of the feet may be cold, atrophic, necrotic or infected depending on the state of the blood supply to the feet. In the upper limbs, Raynaud's phenomenon causes intense vasoconstriction of the fingers and may, in severe cases, progress to gangrene. Unfortunately, none of the vasodilator drugs have been shown to have an appreciable effect in disease states such as these. It is now known that when the arteries are occluded there is little to be gained by attempting to dilate them. Occasionally ischaemic skin ulceration may be helped by the so-called alpha adrenergic blocking agents which relieve vasoconstrictor tone in the skin. Phenoxybenzamine is one of these agents, another is Tolazoline.

Tolazoline

This drug acts on the smooth muscle wall of the arterioles and causes it to relax. Vasodilatation results from this and the blood flow to the part is increased. Tolazoline is usually given orally. It produces best results in patients with Raynaud's phenomenon. It can be given intravenously but is then very liable to cause postural hypotension and the drug is therefore not given intravenously unless the patient is recumbent. A typical dose of tolazoline is 50 mg four times a day by mouth.

4

Drugs used in the treatment of respiratory diseases

In this chapter the antibiotics which are commonly used in treating infective diseases of the respiratory system are not discussed. These drugs are discussed in Chapter 5.

THE TREATMENT OF ASTHMA

In asthmatic patients reversible obstruction in the airways causes wheeze and dyspnoea. This may occur as an allergic response to such stimuli as house dust, to animal fur or may result from emotional stress or respiratory infection. The general management of an asthmatic patient during a severe attack includes the parenteral administration of bronchodilator drugs and corticosteroids, oxygen therapy, removal of the patient from emotional stress and allergic stimuli through admission to hospital. If there is any suspicion of infection broad spectrum antibiotics are given and many physicians prescribe these automatically during an acute attack. Prevention of further attacks involves manipulation of the patient's home environment by the removal of allergic stimuli, help with stressful encounters, and use of the drug sodium chromoglycate which inhibits the body's allergic response to outside stimuli.

Bronchodilator drugs

You will remember from Chapter 3 that the sympathetic nervous system sends fribres to the heart and lungs. These beta adrenergic fibres when stimulated produce an increase in heart rate and a relaxation of the smooth muscle in the bronchioles. When they are blocked by beta adrenergic blocking agents, the reverse occurs, with the resultant slowing of the heart and, in susceptible individuals, bronchospasm. Bronchodilator drugs act by stimulating the adrenergic receptors in the lungs (i.e. they have the opposite action of beta blockers). Some drugs act on both the beta one (cardiac) and beta two (lung) receptors while others act only on the beta two receptors. Most can be administered orally, parenterally or by inhalation.

Adrenaline

This is a time-honoured remedy which was one of the first drugs to be effective in the emergency management of severe asthma (sometimes called status asthmaticus). It is a very potent stimulator of adrenergic receptors in the heart, lungs and blood vessels. In a severe asthmatic attack it is administered subcutaneously. It must not be given intravenously because of the risk of cardiac arrest. A $1/1000$ solution is usually used in a dose of 0.3 to 0.5 ml. Adrenaline may also be administered by inhalation and is included in a number of proprietary aerosols which often contain a number of different bronchodilator drugs. In the management of severe asthma, adrenaline has been superceded by new drugs which are more selective in their action on the lungs and are generally safer.

Isoprenaline

Isoprenaline is an important stimulator of adrenergic receptors in the heart and lungs. It is contained in many aerosol sprays and is effective in this form. Like adrenaline, its parenteral administration carries the risk of producing ventricular arrhythmias and it should not be given by this route in asthma.

The use of isoprenaline aerosols may have been responsible for a number of deaths in asthmatic patients possibly because of overuse of the pressurised dispenser of isoprenaline.

Aminophylline

This is a very useful drug for the emergency treatment of asthma. It acts predominantly on the beta two receptors in the lungs and although it does produce beta stimulation in the heart, this is much less marked than with adrenalin or isoprenaline. Aminophylline is usually administered by slow intravenous injection of 125 to 500 mg in an acute attack, and will often produce rapid improvement. In this situation the drug's action may wear off within an hour or two and as an alternative to the repeated injections aminophylline can be administered by continuous slow intravenous infusion. If aminophylline is injected too rapidly it may produce cardiac arrhythmias. Some individuals seem very sensitive to the drug developing pallor and sweating even after a small intravenous dose. If these features develop while the drug is being injected intravenously it should be discontinued. Aminophylline may be given by an aerosol for the routine treatment of asthma. During more severe attacks it can be delivered by a positive pressure ventilator (Bird Ventilator) which assists the patient's respiratory effort, provides the correct quantity of humidified oxygen and insures that the drug, in the form of fine droplets, reaches the small airways where it produces its beneficial effect. Aminophylline may be given in oral form. Nausea due to gastric irritation is common, although this may be less of a problem with more modern enteric-coated preparations. You will often see aminophylline given in the form of suppositories last thing at night. Some people seem to derive benefit from this procedure although the amount of drug which is absorbed into the blood stream is probably very variable and sometimes very small.

Salbutamol

This is probably the most widely used drug in the management of asthma. Its action is mainly on the beta two adrenergic receptors in the lungs resulting in bronchial dilation without the risk of ventricular arrhythmias. Salbutamol can be given orally when it is absorbed with little gastric irritation. It an also be given subcutaneously or intravenously in the acute attack, and more recently continuous infusions of the drug for up to 24 hours or more have been used successfully in status asthmaticus. Salbutamol is also effective when given by inhaler for the routine management of asthma. Like aminophylline it can be administered by the Bird positive pressure ventilator during severe attack. The usual oral dose of salbutamol is 2 to 4 mg 6-hourly. Tremor is a common side effect when the drug is given orally or parenterally but is not a problem when delivered by inhaler. A simple (sinus) tachy-cardia may be observed in the patients receiving large doses.

Terbutaline

Terbutaline is closely related to salbutamol. It can be adminis-tered by the same routes and has similar side effects.

Miscellaneous bronchodilator drugs

A wide and rather baffling range of bronchodilator drugs is available commercially. They include orciprenaline and ephe-drine. (similar in action to isoprenaline) and theophylline, acepi-fylline and diprophylline (similar in action to aminophylline). These drugs have not been considered individually as they offer no advantage over the commonly used drugs in this section.

Use of bronchodilator aerosols

Administration of brochodilator drugs by aerosol spray has the advantages that high concentrations of the drug are delivered to the lungs while side effects are few because little drug enters the body. Failure of treatment is frequently due to poor inhaler technique. It is very important that you supervise your patient's initial attempts to master his device:

1. Check that the patient is able to compress the device prop-erly.
2. Instruct him to take a deep breath and then *empty his lungs completely.*
3. The mouthpiece is then placed in the mouth and a good seal formed by the lips.
4. The patient then takes a deep breath and *simultaneously* ejects a dose of drug.
5. The breath is held for as long as possible and the patient then breaths out *slowly* through pursed lips.

Corticosteroids in asthma

Corticosteriods are important drugs in the management of asthma. They have no adrenergic stimulant properties but probably act by inhibiting the inflammatory response within the walls of the small airways. In severe asthma, the narrowing of the bronchial walls is caused not only by constriction of this smooth muscle layer but also by inflammatory swelling of the walls and it is here that corticosteroids exert their effect. When administered in acute asthma, corticosteroids take much longer to act than beta adrenergic drugs but once the effect appears, it is much more sustained. If there is any suspicion that an acute severe exacerbation of asthma is not going to respond to simple bronchodilator treatment, corticosteriods must be administered as they are the only drugs which will prove really effective in this situation. There is evidence that preventable deaths from asthma have occurred when these drugs have been administered too late and in insufficient doses.

The naturally occurring compound hydrocortisone is often used in the acute attack administered intravenously in a dose of 100 to 500 mg depending on the urgency of the situation. This is usually followed by a course of oral prednisolone starting with 40 to 60 mg per day in divided doses, steadily reducing and eventually withdrawing the drug over the next 2 to 3 weeks. Patients with asthma of exceptional severity may have to remain on chronic corticosteroid therapy. This should be avoided if possible, especially in children. If it is necessary, the drug should be administered as a single daily dose or on alternate days only, as this reduces the long-term side effects. Like the bronchodilator drugs, corticosteroids can be administered directly to the bronchioles in the form of an inhaler. Beclomethasone—a potent synthetic steroid—is the form frequently used and patients whose asthma cannot be controlled in the long-term by bronchodilator drugs alone can sometimes be helped in this fashion without the dangers of long-term oral steroid therapy. These dangers are discussed fully in a section on Corticosteroid therapy in Chapter 8. A useful tip for patients on steroid inhalers is to take the inhalation 20 to 30 minutes after their last dose of their bronchodilator aerosol, e.g. salbutamol. In this way the bronchodilator drug will have improved their respiratory function and the steroid drug will penetrate better into the small airways.

Sodium Chromoglycate

The main use for sodium chromoglycate is in the *prevention* of asthmatic attacks. The drug is of no value during the acute episode.

Many patients with asthma are allergic to substances such as house dust, cat dander, pollen and certain bacteria. Sodium chromoglycate inhibits the release in the body of histamine and related substances which arise when these allergic patients are exposed to the source of their allergy. The effect of these substances is to cause bronchoconstriction, mediated both by constriction of the smooth muscle in the bronchial wall and also by inflammatory swelling of the bronchial mucosa.

The drug comes as a dry powder in a gelatin capsule. A special device ('Spinhaler') puncture the capsule. The air turbulence caused by the patient's act of inspiration causes the capsule to be spun round and vibrated in the inspired air stream thus ensuring that microscopic particles of powder are inhaled. The dose is 2 to 8 capsules daily; each capsule contains 20 mg of drug.

Oxygen therapy in asthma

Unlike the patient with severe chronic bronchitis the individual with asthma is not usually in a state of chronic hypoxia. In a severe asthmatic attack however bronchoconstriction will greatly reduce ventilation of the small airways and the oxygen level in the blood will fall. Thus those cases which require hospital admission generally benefit from oxygen therapy and in some cases this can be safely given at high concentrations. In more severe prolonged asthmatic attacks the carbon dioxide level of the blood starts to rise and these patients are at risk of respiratory depression if they receive high concentrations of oxygen (see section on oxygen therapy in respiratory failure). It is clear that great care must be taken when administering oxygen to an asthmatic. Estimation of blood gas levels assists the physician in making the correct decision. This is an essential investigation in severe cases. In general you should seek advice regarding the correct concentration before administering oxygen to a patient with asthma.

TREATMENT OF CHRONIC BRONCHITIS

This condition ranges from a mild disorder of the lungs characterised by chronic cough and spit to a severe crippling illness in which the patient is chair-bound with chronic respiratory and cardiac failure. Clearly the management of the individual patient depends on the severity of his condition. Those individuals who are mildly affected may have little incapacity throughout their lives, while others develop features of airways obstruction at an early stage and progress to the more severe forms of the disease. There is overwhelming evidence to link chronic bronchitis with cigarette smoking. This fact must be explained to every patient in an attempt to stop the habit. This is particularly important in younger patients who may have early evidence of airways obstruction or emphysema as the progress of their disease can be slowed or even halted. Clearly cessation of smoking is all that is required in mild cases. A wide range of drugs is used in patients with chronic bronchitis including bronchodilators, antibacterial drugs and diuretics. The question of oxygen therapy and respiratory stimulants will be considered under the management of respiratory failure.

Bronchodilators in chronic bronchitis

Bronchodilator drugs have been considered fully in the section on asthma. In chronic bronchitis with obstructive features the same drugs are used. It is important to realise that in chronic bronchitis much of the obstruction is irreversible and therefore may be refractory to drug treatment. An attempt should be made using breathing tests to assess the patient's ability to respond to drugs such as aminophylline, salbutamol, and corticosteroids. If a response is apparent then these drugs should be used. Clearly, when obstruction of small airways is due to retention of viscid sputum, chest physiotherapy is of vital importance and is more effective than any drug therapy.

Antibacterial drugs

Chronic bronchitis is not primarily an infective condition. With chronic airways obstruction and overproduction of sputum, however, sufferers are very likely to develop infection following common colds and flu. The common infecting organisms are *Pneumococcus* and *Haemophilus influenzae*. Broad spectrum antibiotics such as ampicillin, co-trimoxazole and cephalosporins are commonly used during these exacerbations. If the sputum appears to be purulent, the broad spectrum penicillin derivatives are probably the drugs of choice as they are always effective against the two organisms mentioned. There is no evidence that long-term treatment with antibiotics is of any benefit to patients with chronic bronchitis as they do not halt the progress of this disease. The antibaterial drugs in common use are considered in greater detail in Chapter 5.

Diuretics and digoxin

Patients with severe chronic bronchitis and pulmonary hypertension may develop cardiac failure. This condition is known as cor pulmonale and the discovery of potent diuretics such as frusemide and the aldosterone antagonist spironolactone has greatly improved the outlook of patients with this condition. Diuretic drugs are considered in greater detail in Chapter 3. There is some argument about the benefits of digoxin in cor pulmonale as most cases remain in sinus rhythm. Many physicians restrict its use to the most severe cases.

MANAGEMENT OF RESPIRATORY FAILURE

Respiratory failure is said to occur when oxygenation of blood in the lungs is insufficient to meet the needs of the body. In practice this means that the oxygen level in the blood is low and in many cases the carbon dioxide level is elevated. Obviously respiratory failure may result from a wide range of causes, including inhalation of carbon monoxide, respiratory centre depression by drug overdose, severe pneumonia, pulmonary embolus, severe asthma and chronic bronchitis and emphysema. The last cause is by far the commonest. In severe chronic bronchitis, the irreversible airways obstruction leads to chronic respiratory failure with low oxygen and elevated carbon dioxide levels. Patients manage remarkably well despite this but in acute exacerbations with infection in the airways, further obstruction due to retention of purulent sputum occurs and the patient may quickly become moribund and comatose. At this stage profound hypoxia, severe carbon dioxide poisoning and acidosis threaten life. This situation requires prompt treatment. The successful treatment of respiratory failure depends on the maintenance of a clear airway and vigorous aspiration of retained secretions. In severe cases intubation and mechanical ventilatory assistance may be required although careful thought must be given to this decision because of the difficulty often encountered in 'weaning off' such patients later.

Oxygen therapy in respiratory failure

Although it may be possible to give high concentrations of oxygen to patients with acute pulmonary oedema or pneumonia, patients with respiratory failure resulting from chronic bronchitis or severe prolonged asthma are a separate group due to the high concentrations of carbon dioxide in the blood. If high concentrations of oxygen are administered to these patients there is the risk of further accumulation of carbon dioxide in the blood stream leading to the condition of carbon dioxide narcosis. It is important that you have a clear grasp of how this condition arises, which patients are liable to develop it and how to prevent this complication arising in susceptible subjects. A knowledge of the chemical factors controlling respiration is helpful in understanding how CO_2 narcosis comes about.

The respiratory centre normally stimulates the lungs to inspire when the level of CO_2 in the blood reaches a certain critical level. When the lungs expire, this critical blood level of CO_2 is reduced because CO_2 is exhaled. The respiratory centre therefore stops stimulating the lungs to inspire and it is not until the blood level of CO_2 again reaches the critical level that the cycle repeats itself. You should read this paragraph again to obtain a clear image of the normal situation before proceeding to the description of the abnormal situation.

In some patients with long-standing chronic bronchitis and emphysema, the disease process in the lungs renders it difficult for the lungs to excrete CO_2. In these patient's blood chronically high levels of CO_2 are established. Initially the respiratory centre breathes more quickly because of the high level of CO_2 in the blood (just as a normal person does when given 5 per cent CO_2 to inhale from a cylinder). After a time, however, the respiratory centre ceases to be stimulated by the high blood levels of CO_2 and becomes used to these levels. This means that CO_2 now plays no part in stimulating these patients to breathe. What then does stimulate the respiratory centre of some patients with chronic bronchitis and emphysema? The answer is lack of oxygen in the blood (known as hypoxia). During expiration the blood level of oxygen starts to fall and when it reaches a critically low level the respiratory centre becomes activated and stimulates inspiration. Oxygen is then inhaled, the blood oxygen level rises, the activity of the respiratory centre ceases and expiration begins. The oxygen level in the blood starts to fall once more and at the critically low level the respiratory centre is again activated producing inspiration. This state of affairs is not satisfactory because breathing is inefficient and these patients are chronically anoxic. If, however, you give them oxygen to breathe in high concentrations, the blood oxygen level becomes very high and the respiratory centre is no longer stimulated. The patients rapidly breathe more and more shallowly until they may stop breathing altogether and die in coma. The term CO_2 narcosis is applied to this coma. You can see that it has been induced by oxygen therapy. Yet these patients *need* oxygen. How are these two seemingly contradictory situations to be resolved?

The most satisfactory solution is to give oxygen at a low concentration in the inspired air. This very gently and slowly corrects the blood and tissue oxygen deficit but does not cause inhibition of the respiratory centre. There are special masks for delivering oxygen at a low concentration in the inspired air and these are used to give oxygen to patients in whom the danger of CO_2 narcosis is anticipated.

Shortly after the introduction of oxygen therapy for resuscitating premature babies, it was found that many of these infants later became blind. By a brilliant piece of research work Professor Norman Ashton was able to show the cause of this blindness and better still how to prevent it. He took baby kittens and exposed them to high concentrations of oxygen. He found that when he killed the kittens and examined their eyes a white sheet of fibrous tissue was growing over the retina. The tissue which was opaque to light was making the kittens blind. The term for this condition is retrolental fibroplasia which means a growth of fibrous tissue behind the lens. Ashton demonstrated that if the oxygen concentration in the inspired air was less than 40 per cent, retrolental fibroplasia did not develop. Thanks to this work many premature infants have been spared a lifetime of blindness.

Methods of administration of oxygen

Before administering oxygen to a patient it is essential to determine what concentration is required. This will not be your decision, so make a point of immediately asking the medical staff responsible for the case when oxygen is required for any patient under your care. Nowadays oxygen is always administered to adult patients by some form of face mask or device. Oxygen tents are no longer used as they are extremely inefficient, inconveni-

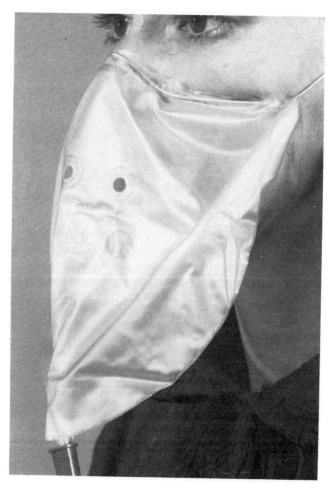

Fig. 4.1 Polymask

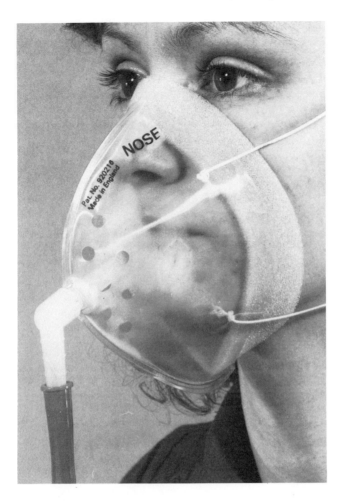

Fig. 4.2 MC mask

ent and are a fire risk. A number of face masks are in common
use. They vary in the concentration of oxygen supplied to the
patient. When a high flow mask is needed (40 to 60 per cent
oxygen) the oxygen will be dry and it is essential that some form
of humidifying device is used.

Polymask (Fig. 4.1). This is a simple cheap mask which delivers
high concentrations of oxygen only. The oxygen flow rate should
be kept at 8 litres per minute when using this mask. Obviously it
should never be used to treat patients with carbon dioxide

narcosis as the high oxygen levels may lead to respiratory depression. This mask has no rigid frame and if the oxygen supply is turned off the mask may collapse around the patient's mouth and nose with the danger of asphyxia.

The MC mask (Fig. 4.2). The concentration of oxygen delivered by this mask depends on the oxygen flow rate. At rates in excess of 4 litre per minute it provides a concentration of 40 per cent although this varies from patient to patient. It should not be used by patients with carbon dioxide retention.

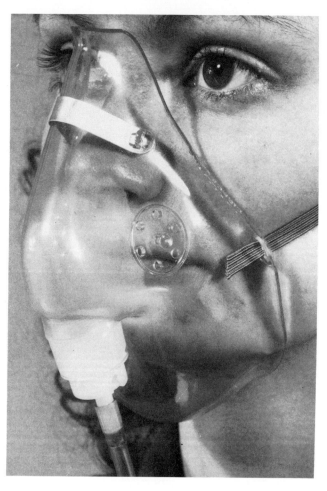

Fig. 4.3 Hudson mask

The Hudson Mask (Fig. 4.3). Like the MC mask the oxygen concentration will depend on the flow rate, but it is nearly always used to deliver high concentration (40 to 60 per cent) and should not be given to patients with carbon dioxide retention.

Ventimask (Fig. 4.4). This is the most popular mask for patients who require low oxygen concentrations (24 to 28 per cent) for treatment of respiratory failure caused by chronic bronchitis. The performance of this mask is fixed. This means that it will deliver the same concentration of oxygen to the patient irrespec-

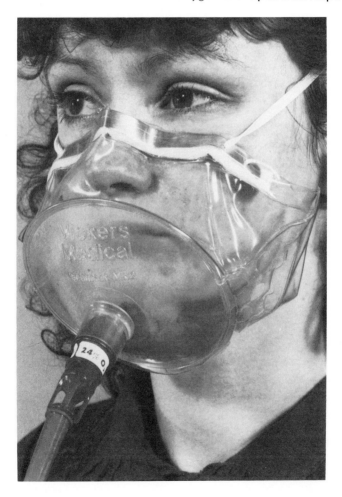

Fig. 4.4 Ventimask

tive of the oxygen flow rate. Several versions of the mask are available but you will see the 24 and 28 per cent models in routine use.

Mix-o-mask (Fig. 4.5). Like the Ventimask this device has a fixed performance and is designed to deliver oxygen at lower concentrations for the treatment of patients with chronic obstructive lung disease. Both 24 and 28 per cent versions are available and are used in an identical fashion to the older Ventimask. Other versions of this mask deliver higher concentra-

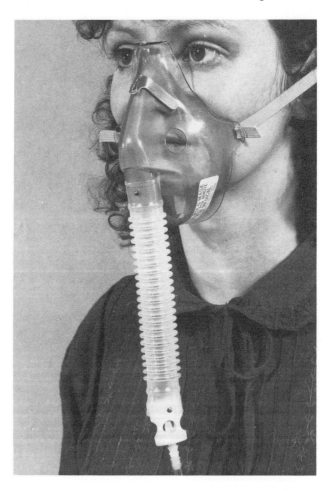

Fig. 4.5 Mix-o-mask

tions (up to 40 per cent oxygen). As with the Ventimask it is essential that you establish that the patient has been given the correct model which delivers the precise concentration of oxygen that he or she requires.

Nasal Carnulae. This device is not a mask but a simple duplicated nasal catheter one end of which is placed in each nostril. They are not really suitable for patients with nasal blockage, but have the advantage that they are comfortable and are more likely to be tolerated by agitated or confused patients. The oxygen concentration depends on the flow rate, but at low rates (1 to 2 litres per min) they can be used to treat patients with carbon dioxide narcosis provided they are very closely observed.

Nursing observations to be made on patients receiving oxygen therapy

1. Ensure that no patients in the vicinity are smoking or have access to matches.
2. Make sure that the mask is applied firmly to your patient's face and that he can tolerate it readily.
3. Check the flow rate of oxygen every hour or so.
4. In patients with chronic bronchitis and emphysema watch for signs of worsening respiratory failure. These are deepening cyanosis while on oxygen; gradual diminution in rate of respiration (which should be counted regularly) or gradual loss of consciousness.

Respiratory stimulants in respiratory failure

The use of respiratory stimulants is a controversial subject and many physicians believe they have little to offer in the treatment of respiratory failure. When a patient's respiration is so depressed that they are at risk of dying then the correct management is intubation of the trachea and mechanical ventilation. When dealing with a patient suffering from chronic lung disease it may be decided that the individual is not suitable for this type of ventilatory assistance because of the chronic and severe nature of the condition, and the fact that it may not be possible to discontinue mechanical ventilation once the acute phase of the illness is past. The decision whether or not to provide mechanical assistance to a patient with chronic lung disease is always a very difficult one. Such factors as their previous history, the severity of the disease while it is in remission and the quality of their life prior to admission are all taken into account. In a case like this the short-term use of respiratory stimulants is probably correct as it may help to support the individual through an acute deterioration in respiratory function. These drugs in general have little direct effect on respiration but tend to increase the patient's conscious level and allow the return of the cough reflex and improve expectoration of sputum.

Nikethimide

This drug has been in use for a long time but is still occasionally used to resuscitate a patient with severe respiratory failure. In this situation it is usually given intravenously and may be combined in an injection with aminophylline. The effect of the drug is to increase the general level of arousal. Precipitation of full blown epileptic seizures is a very real risk if the drug is given too quickly or in large doses. Muscular twitching is commonly observed during the injection.

Aminophylline

It is not widely known but this drug and other members of the theophylline group have a mild stimulant action on the respiratory centre and this may be of use in respiratory failure.

Doxapram

This is a relatively new drug and seems to have a genuine stimulant effect on the respiratory centre. It can be given by the intramuscular route but in respiratory failure is usually administered as a constant infusion which is adjusted to deliver the smallest dose which is required to maintain adequate respiration. Side effects of this drug are excessive restlessness, tremor, tachycardia and in susceptible individuals, seizures.

Cough suppressants

A number of drugs are available which genuinely depress the cough reflex by central action on the medulla. These drugs are commonly prescribed for common coughs and colds but in general, suppression of cough reflex is not a desirable aim in patients with chronic respiratory disease. Occasionally, intractable cough develops as a symptom in a patient with inoperable lung cancer. These patients are always treated very vigorously with powerful cough suppressants as respiratory depression is not a major worry.

Codeine phosphate

This drug is usually given in the form of a syrup when it is being used as a cough suppressant. Syrup of codeine phosphate is a pleasant tasting mixture and it can be given to children in the knowledge that this is one medicine that they will like. Most of them, in fact, ask for more. Many firms which manufacture drugs make their own cough suppressants. If you read the label on their bottles you will often discover that the active ingredient is codeine. As proprietary preparations of medicine tend to be twice to ten times or more as expensive as medicines which are officially approved, syrup of codeine phosphate is to be preferred to these other preparations.

Those of you who make your career in nursing outside hospital will often be called upon to advise on the correct dosage of this drug. For adults an average-sized dose of syrup of codeine phosphate is two teaspoonfuls four times a day. (The average teaspoon holds 4 ml. Two teaspoonfuls of the preparation corresponds to approximately 24 mg of codeine.) For children less than a year old one quarter of a teaspoonful made up to a whole teaspoonful with water should be given not more than three times a day. Children between 1 and 3 years of age receive a half-teaspoonful, children between 3 and 5 years, three-quarters of a teaspoonful and children between 5 and 12 a whole teaspoonful, not more than three times a day.

Codeine has other actions. It is an analgesic and is used in the treatment of diarrhoea. These aspects of its use are discussed more fully in Chapter 7. Many patients treated with codeine become constipated as a side effect of the drug.

Morphine and its derivatives

Occasionally it is necessary to suppress a cough for palliative reasons. For example a patient with an inoperable bronchogenic carcinoma may experience a racking non-productive cough which does not respond to codeine. In these situations morphine or one of its closer derivatives such as methadone or physeptone is of utmost value. Methadone is commonly used for the purpose in the form linctus methadone (linctus means syrup). One is normally cautious about giving morphine or its derivatives on a long-term basis because of the fear of producing addiction in a patient who is going to recover from his illness at a later date. This consideration does not apply when patients with inoperable carcinoma are being treated.

Sedative drugs in respiratory failure

You will note that the drugs used for suppression of cough also depress respiration. This is a grave risk in a patient with chronic lung disease and respiratory failure and almost completely prevents the prescription of cough suppressants for such patients. It is vital that you appreciate that patients with chronic lung disease are very sensitive to the effects of *all* sedative drugs. Potent respiratory depressants such as morphine are the greatest risk but even a small dose of diazepam or dihydrocodeine (DF. 118) may be enough to tip a patient into acute respiratory failure. All of these drugs must be avoided if at all possible.

Expectorants

An expectorant is a substance which increases the production of sputum. As has been discussed in the previous section, if mucus is produced in the bronchi and bronchioles, it must be cleared from the lungs by coughing. In some patients, however, the mucus is viscid and tenacious and it is extremely difficult for these patients to produce sputum. Before, many drugs were thought to be good expectorants and were used widely in clinical practice to help clear away this kind of mucus. There is no doubt that these substances did cause the patient to produce sputum, but we now realise that they did this by stimulating the bronchi and bronchioles to produce fresh liquid sputum which was easily coughed up. The viscid sputum remained stuck fast in the bronchi. Only one of these widely used remedies has stood the test of time and it is still used today. It is a simple remedy and extremely efficient in helping the patient rid himself of viscid mucus: steam.

Steam inhalations

It might seem odd to you that a simple remedy such as inhaling steam is of value as an expectorant. The reason for its great value is that steam is inhaled *as a gas* and therefore it can pass with ease down the smallest bronchioles to the site of obstruction by mucus. It then becomes water which helps moisten and soften the tenacious mucus thus making it easier for the patient to dislodge the plug.

Many patients are quite frankly a bit sceptical of the value of this simple remedy. To impress them somewhat more and to ensure that they practise their inhalations if they are at home, menthol crystals are often added to the recipe. Menthol crystals have an extremely pungent and penetrating odour and to the lay person they smell extremely health-giving. However, they add nothing to the expectorant effect of the steam inhalation.

Technique of administering a steam inhalation. Many of you who practise outside hospital will have to advise your patients how to assemble a steam inhalation. To the bottom of a tall jug add three to four menthol crystals. Fill the jug two-thirds full with boiling water. Instruct your patient to cover the top of the jug with a towel and, using the towel as a mask, to inhale the vapours through it. If a towel is not used there is a risk of your patient scalding his face on the hot steam.

Antihistamines

Antihistamine drugs are used in a wide variety of conditions but most commonly in disorders of the upper respiratory tract. For this reason their inclusion in the chapter on respiratory diseases is appropriate. The antihistamine group contains a wide variety of drugs which all, to a greater or lesser extent, antagonise some of the actions of histamine. The histamine receptors in the nose, respiratory tract and skin, can be blocked by these compounds but they have no effect on the receptors in the stomach with are responsible for simulating secretion of hydrochloric acid. A completely different drug is required for this, the H_2 receptor antagonist cimetidine (see Chapter 2). The antihistamines are used for the treatment of urticaria, angioneurotic oedema and hay fever. These conditions are all brought about by the action of histamine. In general the drugs are only moderately effective and in hay fever, sodium chromoglycate and corticosteroids by inhalation produce much greater relief. Examples of the antihistamine group of drugs are: mepyramine, diphenhydramine, chlorpheniramine. These drugs are relatively short-acting and have to be given several times a day. By comparison, promethazine, which is related to the phenothiazine group of drugs is long-acting and is usually given once daily before bed. There is little to choose between these drugs as they all tend to produce drowsiness. Indeed, any of them can be used as a gentle hypnotic. This fact plus their tendency to produce dizziness and blurring of vision makes them potentially dangerous as they are often consumed by patients suffering from minor ailments who may be responsible for driving or operating machinery at work. Patients should always be warned about the effects which will be much greater if the drugs are mixed with alcohol.

5

Drugs used in the treatment of infectious diseases

ANTIBIOTICS AND CHEMOTHERAPEUTIC AGENTS

Before discussing the actions of antibiotics and chemotherapeutic agents a few definitions may be helpful.

A chemotherapeutic agent is a *chemically synthesised substance* which is antagonistic to micro-organisms.

An antibiotic is a substance *derived from a living organism* which is antagonistic to the growth or life of other micro-organisms.

Antibiotics were initially developed from colonies of certain fungi or bacteria. These colonies produced substances which would kill or inhibit the growth of other fungi or bacteria which caused some infectious diseases. With the development of new chemical and pharmaceutical techniques it has become possible to synthesise many of these substances in the laboratory without the help of micro-organisms.

Thus the distinction between an antibiotic and a chemotherapeutic agent has become less clear cut than it was formerly.

A bacteriocidal agent is one which *kills* bacteria.

A bacteriostatic agent is one which does not kill bacteria but *halts their multiplication.*

None of the antibiotics or chemotherapeutic agents would be of much value in the treatment of infectious diseases were it not for the great ability of the polymorphonuclear leucocytes to phagocytose bacteria. The antibiotic and chemotherapeutic drugs which are given to the patient with an infection only help the polymorphonuclear leucocytes in fighting and killing bacteria. If the patient has no polymorphs in his blood it is doubtful if any antibiotic can do much to save him. This is why agranulocytosis is such an extremely dangerous and often fatal condition.

In theory you might expect that bacteriocidal agents which kill bacteria would be preferable to bacteriostatic agents which prevent increase in bacterial numbers. In practice there is not a great deal of difference between the two. However, when treating severe infection in a cricially ill patient, most doctors given a choice between employing a bacteriocidal agent or a bacteriostatic one will pick the former. This seems a wise decision.

This chapter will describe the more commonly used chemotherapeutic agents and antibiotics under the following headings: the sulphonamides, the penicillins and cephalosporins, the aminoglycosides, the tetracyclines, the macrolides and lincomycin group, miscellaneous antibiotics and antifungal agents.

Mode of action of antibiotics and chemotherapeutic agents

These drugs act in one of three possible ways although sometimes one agent may act in more than one way.

1. Interference with synthesis of the cell wall of the micro-organism (for example penicillins and cephalosporins).
2. Interference with protein synthesis in the micro-organism (for example tetracyclines and aminoglycosides).
3. Interference with metabolism of the micro-organism (for example suphonamides).

SULPHONAMIDES

Sulphonamides were introduced into clinical practice in 1935. They were discovered after a great deal of work had been done on the action of certain dyes (for example gentian violet) in killing bacteria. The problem was that while some dyes could be shown to be extremely efficient at killing bacteria when they were applied locally to the skins of laboratory animals they killed both bacteria and laboratory animals if given internally. The inference from these experiments was, of course, that these dyes would also kill patients if given internally. It seemed that this was a side effect of treatment which few patients would gladly accept and therefore a search was made for other dyes with antibacterial effects which could be safely given to patients. The dye fitting these requirements was prontosil rubrum. From this compound, the first sulphonamide, sulphapyridine, was developed. There are now a great variety of different sulphonamides available. Six commonly used ones are sulphadimidine, sulphadiazine, sulphafurazole, sulphamethoxazole, phthalylsulphathiazole and sulphasalazine. There is not a great deal to choose between any of these drugs and so it is not necessary for you to know about each one in detail. If you understand the principles behind the use of one sulphonamide these principles can be applied to other sulphomaides. These drugs all act by interfering with the metabolism of folic acid in bacteria.

Sulphadimidine is an excellent sulphonamide for routine use and will be described in detail.

Sulphadimidine

This drug, like the other sulphonamides, is a chemotherapeutic agent and is bacteriostatic. It is usually given orally but can be administered by intravenous injection if the patient is unconscious or too ill to take drugs by mouth. Sulphadimidine, like all sulphonamides, must **never** be given intrathecally. The drug is a strongly irritant substance and sets up an intense inflammatory reaction in the coverings of the spinal cord. This can cause the patient to become paralysed.

Sulphadimidine is usually given in a loading dose of 2 to 3 g to saturate the patient with the drug. A maintenance dose of 1 to 1.5 g is given therafter every 6 hours.

Indications for sulphadimidine

Sulphadimidine is active against a wide variety of bacteria. With the advent of antibiotics the indications for the use of this drug have become less. Generally speaking it is used to treat a patient with an infection which is sensitive only or chiefly to sulphonamides. You will commonly see this drug employed in two clinical conditions: urinary tract infections and meningococcal meningitis. The drug is used in urinary tract infections because the commonly occurring urinary tract pathogen, *E. Coli*, is often sensitive to it. Sulphadimidine is useful in the treatment of meningococcal meningitis because virtually all meningococci are sensitive to its action and also because the drug crosses the blood-brain barrier with ease.

The blood-brain barrier is a curious phenomenon. No one has actually ever demonstrated the anatomical existence of a barrier between the blood and the brain. However, most drugs and many other substances too for that matter, behave as if there were a barrier which prevented them from passing from the blood into the cerebrospinal fluid. Much higher concentrations of penicillin, for example (another drug which is active against meningococci), are found in the blood than in the cerebrospinal fluid. This is not the case with sulphadimidine. The concentration of this drug in the cerebrospinal fluid is equal to its concentration in the blood. In meningococcal meningitis, as you know, meningococci are present in very large numbers in the cerebrospinal fluid. Sulphadimidine is thus able to go to the part of the body where it can do most good.

Side effects of sulphadimidine

Sulphadimidine shares with other sulphonamide drugs the liability to cause four side effects.

1. Anorexia, nausea and vomiting
2. Skin rashes and drug fever
3. Crystalluria
4. Agranulocytosis.

Sulphadimidine may be strongly irritant to the gastric mucosa and many patients feel nauseated after taking the drug by mouth. For this reason it is a useful procedure to try to give sulphadimidine after, rather than before, meals.

Skin rashes of all grades of severity may develop in sensitive individuals taking sulphadimidine. Most rashes are mild but occasionally the dangerous condition exfoliative dermatitis may ensue. An interesting though unusual skin reaction which some subjects develop while taking sulphonamides is photosensitisation of the skin. Quite severe sunburn may occur on exposure to mild sunlight even in patients who have previously prided themselves on their ability to take a good suntan. This side effect constitutes a clear indication for stopping the drug.

Crystalluria, or the passage of crystals of sulphadimidine in the urine after their precipitation into the substance of the kidney, is a possible hazard. This phenomenon is fortunately rare with the modern sulphonamides in use at the present time but was a not-infrequent complication of treatment with earlier sulphonamides. Advising your patient to take a high fluid intake (3 litres per day) to ensure a large urine volume and rendering the urine alkaline, are two measures which help keep sulphadimidine in solution in the urine and minimise the risk of developing crystalluria.

Agranulocytosis (depression of the white cell count is the blood) is a very rare side effect of this and other sulphonamides.

Sulphasalazine

This drug is actually a combination of a sulphonamide and salicylic acid. It is used principally in the treatment of patients with ulcerative colitis. A feeling of nausea is very commonly experienced by patients taking this drug, although it is less of a problem if the total daily dose is kept to 4 g or less. (See Ch. 2).

Co-trimoxazole

This is a combination of sulphamethoxazole (400 mg) with trimethoprin (80 mg) an agent which also interferes with folic acid metabolism in bacteria but in a different way from the sulphonamides.

The combination is bacteriocidal and under the names Bactrim and Septrin is widely used. It is a particularly useful agent for the treatment of urinary and respiratory tract infections, and is more effective than sulphadimidine in the treatment of *E. coli,* the common infecting organism.

The dose is two tablets twice daily.

PENICILLINS

The penicillins are chemically related members of a family of which the parent substance is the antibiotic penicillin. The penicillins are bacteriocidal.

Penicillin

Penicillin was discovered by Sir Alexander Fleming, the Scottish bacteriologist, in 1929. It was not until 1940 that this antibiotic was synthesised and introduced into clinical practice. Penicillin, the first discovered antibiotic, is still today the best all-round antibiotic.

This drug is effective against haemolytic streptococci, *Strep. viridans* pneumococci, gonococci, meningococci, the anthrax bacillus, the organism which causes diptheria (*Corynebacterium diphtheriae*) and the causative organism in syphilis (*Treponema pallidum*). This list (which it is not necessary for you to memorise) will give you an indication of the number of different diseases in which penicillin may be effective. An increasing problem in hospital practice is the growing numbers of bacteria which are developing resistance to penicillin and to other antibiotics. Not long ago the list of organisms which penicillin kills would have included *Staphylococcus aureus*. It is nowadays almost certain that if a patient becomes infected with *Staphylococcus aureus* in hospital, the organism will be resistant to the action of penicillin.

Penicillins act by interfering with synthesis of the cell wall of micro-organisms.

Preparations of penicillin

Benzylpenicillin and procaine benzylpenicillin which are administered parenterally and phenoxymethylpenicillin and phenethicillin which are given orally may all be regarded as different preparations of penicillin. If a patient is to be treated for serious infections one of the two parenteral. preparations must be given by intramuscular or intravenous injection. Benzylpenicillin is usually given as one million units initially, followed by half a million units 6-hourly, although in serious situations, for instance treatment of meningitis or infective endocarditis, doses in the range of 12 to 20 million units per day may be administered. The length of treatment is dictated by the illness being treated and the patient's response to the drug. Procaine benzylpenicillin is a longer acting form of penicillin and it is possible to obtain antibacterial blood levels of this drug for 24 hours following a single injection. Phenoxymethyl penicillin (Penicillin V) is the best oral form of penicillin. Even its absorption is not particularly good and its use is reserved for the treatment of less serious infections such as pharyngitis. Ideally it should be administered on an empty stomach to ensure optimal absorption. The usual dose is 250 to 500 mg 6-hourly.

Side effects of penicillin

Penicillin may rarely cause severe and sometimes fatal sensitivity reactions after its use (penicillin allergy). Milder reactions take the form of fever, skin rashes and transient attacks of pain and swelling in the joints. More severe reactions can cause hypotensive collapse which may lead to death.

Penicillin should *never* be given to patients who have had reactions to it in the past. In these patients further exposure to penicillin may cause death. Each year a number of people die following the effects of an injection or series of injections of penicillin. It has been estimated that probably half of these lives could have been saved had the doctor or nurse, before injecting penicillin, asked the simple question, 'Have you ever had any kind of upset such as a fever or skin rash after a penicillin injection?' If a patient *has* had such a side effect he is very liable to know all about it. Therefore if he says 'no' to this question it is safe to proceed.

You should note that rashes with ampicillin are much more common than with benzylpenicillin and if the patient has a history of this it does not necessarily mean that he or she will develop a serious allergy to benzylpenicillin. Obviously in less serious situations an alternative drug must be used, but if benzylpenicillin is essential, for instance in the treatment of meningitis or endocarditis, it should never be withheld because of a history of ampicillin sensitivity. In this situation a small test dose of benezylpenicillin should be given and if there is no reaction to this full doses can be administered.

Cloxacillin, and Flucloxacillin

These members of the penicillin family are not as active against bacteria as is ordinary penicillin. They have the great advantage that they can be used to treat patients with infections caused by strains of the *Staphylococcus aureus* which are resistant to benzylpenicillin and its related preparations, procaine ben-zylpenicillin and phenoxymethylpenicillin. You will notice that in clinical practice the use of cloxacillin and flucloxaccilin is restricted to the treatment of severely ill patients with infections caused by penicillin-resistant staphylococci. The drugs may be given by intramuscular injection in a dose of 250 mg 6-hourly. The injection is painful and if it is necessary to continue treat-ment when the patient is on the road to recovery, cloxacillin or flucloxacillin may be given orally at that stage. Flucloxacillin has the advantage of being particularly well absorbed after oral administration.

Carbenicillin

Carbenicillin is a penicillin derivative which is particularly active against an organism known as pseudomonas which is resistant to other penicillins and indeed many other antibiotics. It is given in a dose of 2 to 5 g 4 to 6-hourly by intramuscular or intravenous injection. This drug is now becoming less popular following the widespread availability of alternatives such as the aminoglyco-side group of antibiotics.

BROAD SPECTRUM PENICILLINS

Ampicillin

This member of the penicillin family has no action against penic-illin-resistant staphylococci. It is very active, however, against a wide range of Gram-negative bacilli which are not sensitive to penicillin. Ampicillin is useful in the treatment of some urinary tract infections and is particularly popular for treatment of respiratory infections involving the organism *Haemophilus influenzae*. The drug may be given orally or by intramuscular injection in a dose of 250 to 500 mg four times a day.

Side effects of ampicillin

The most common side effect of ampicillin therapy is a rash, which develops in around 8 per cent of patients. If the drug is given mistakenly for a viral illness, and particularly in glandular fever, rashes can be very common indeed. Diarrhoea and fungal infections of the oropharynx are a problem with this and all broad spectrum antibiotics and are due to changes in the normal bacterial flora in these areas.

Amoxycillin

Amoxycillin has a similar spectrum of action to ampicillin but has the advantage of being much better absorbed after oral administration. Higher levels of the drug in the blood stream are therefore achieved with a smaller dose. The usual dose is 250 mg 8-hourly.

THE CEPHALOSPORINS

These are antibiotics derived from the cephalosporin mould. Like penicillin they act by interfering with the bacterial cell wall. They are broad spectrum antibiotics with a range of antibacterial activity approximately equal to ampicillin, and in addition some are active against staphylococci resistant to benzylpenicillin.

Patients who are allergic to penicillin are sometimes, but not always, allergic to the cephalosporins. The chief use of these agents is in the treatment of penicillin-resistant staphylocci and the treatment of patients with Gram-negative infections of the urinary tract. Cephalosporins are not as effective as ampicillin against *Haemophilus influenzae,* the common infecting organism in chronic bronchitis. As a group, they are not particularly well absorbed from the gastrointestinal tract and most have to be injected.

Cephaloridine

Parenteral administration of cephaloridine is necessary because the drug is not absorbed orally. Intramuscular injection can be painful.

Cephaloridine may cause renal damage and this is more likely to happen if the kidneys are already diseased or if the patient is concurrently receiving diuretic therapy.

The dose is usually 250 to 1000 mg 6-hourly

Cephalothin

This drug is similar to cephaloridine but may cause less renal damage.

Cephalexin

This member of the family of cephalosporins is active when given orally. The dose is 250 mg 6-hourly. It is not so effective as the other members against *Staph. aureas*.

THE AMINOGLYCOSIDES

This group of powerful antibiotics is derived from naturally occurring fungi. They have a spectrum of potent bacteriocidal activity against a wide range of organisms including *E. coli*, Klebsiella, Entrobacter, *Staphylococcus aureas* and *Mycobacterium tuberculosis*. They act by inhibiting bacterial protein synthesis. They are not absorbed from the gut and must be injected. Their use should be reserved for life-threatening systemic infections, particularly when the nature of the infecting organism is not known in the early stages of treatment. All of these drugs tend to produce serious side effects, notably damage to the kidneys and to the eighth (vestibulocochlear) nerve, resulting in vertigo or deafness.

Streptomycin

Streptomycin is a bacteriocidal antibiotic which was first isolated in 1944 from the *Streptomyces griseus* and it is from this fungus that it derives its name.

Streptomycin is particularly active agains the tubercle bacillus. Its main role has been in the treatment of tuberculosis and its use in this situation is discussed in the section on antituberculous drugs. In the past it was also used in a wide range of other infectious conditions but is now less popular as alternative drugs have become available which are less toxic.

Side effects of streptomycin

There are two main side effects of streptomycin.

1. Skin rashes
2. Damage to both parts of the eighth cranial nerve.

Skin rashes. It is very important that you know about the liability of streptomycin to cause contact dermatitis for this is an action of the drug which affects not only the patient but the nurse. Many nurses who work regularly with streptomycin in tuberculosis wards develop an intractible contact dermatitis of the hands. A few nurses have had to change their interests to another branch of nursing because of this side effect. Occasionally the condition occurs in susceptible nurses who had been exposed only briefly to the drug in general medical or surgical wards. It is a wise precaution to wear gloves when administering streptomycin and you should avoid spraying fine droplets of the drug into the air when you are expelling air from your syringe.

Eighth cranial nerve damage. This is a very serious side effect of streptomycin treatment. You will recall that the fibres of the eighth cranial nerve subserve the faculty of hearing and are in part responsible for the maintenance of balance. It is this latter function of the nerve which is principally damaged by streptomycin, resulting in loss of balance. If this becomes severe it is likely to be irreversible when the drug is stopped. Deafness may also occur in patients receiving streptomycin.

Streptomycin is excreted by the kidneys and in patients with inpaired kidney function high blood levels of the drug are maintained for a long period. This is particularly liable to induce damage to the eighth cranial nerve. Dehydrated patients are also likely to develop high blood levels of streptomycin. You should therefore ensure that all of your patients receiving treatment with streptomycin have a liberal fluid intake. It is especially important to do this in old and in febrile patients.

Gentamicin

This is the most commonly prescribed aminoglycoside antibiotic in hospitals in the United Kingdom. It has a very broad spectrum of action and is particularly effective against pseudomonas and coliform organisms. This has made it the first choice antibiotic for treatment of life-threatening infections in hospital. The main risks associated with its use are damage to the vestibular nerve and the kidneys. Toxicity can be reduced by careful control of dosage, which must be reduced when renal impairment is suspected. As an aid to therapy the blood level of this and other aminoglycoside drugs is often measured during therapy. This helps to avoid toxicity associated with high concentrations of the drug and also ensures that enough is present in the blood to be effective. The usual dose of gentamicin is 80 mg 8-hourly but this must be guided by measurements of renal function and drug concentrations in the blood.

Tobramycin

This drug is more popular outside the United Kingdom. It has similar properties to gentamicin and is used in the same clinical situations. It may be less likely to produce kidney damage but as yet this has not been definitely proven.

Kanamycin

This drug is now little used as gentamicin is more effective. One situation where it is still popular is in the treatment of gonorrhoea where a single intramuscular injection will eradicate infection.

Neomycin

This drug is too toxic for parenteral administration. It is reserved for sterilisation of the intestine when it is usually given in a dose of 1 to 2 g 6-hourly. It is most frequently used for sterilisation of the bowel prior to surgery and is also used in patients with hepatic coma to reduce the production of toxic nitrogenous products by bacteria in the bowel. It is not absorbed in significant quantities following oral administration but in renal failure enough drug may accumulate in the body to damage the eighth cranial nerve.

TETRACYCLINES

This group of chemotherapeutic agents has been available for a long time but the advent of more effective antibiotic drugs has lessened their importance. They have a fairly wide spectrum of action but they are bacteriostatic agents of fairly low potency and tend not to be fully absorbed from the gut. They should not be used in life-threatening systemic infections. One valuable aspect of their activity is their effectiveness against a group of unusual organisms including mycoplasma (primary atypical pneumonia), rickettsiae (Q-fever) and the psittacosis group. These organisms are not susceptible to other antibacterial drugs and the tetracyclines remain the drugs of first choice for treatment of these conditions.

Tetracyclines are also used for the treatment of brucellosis and in low doses are effective in acne vulgaris. A wide variety of agents is available but it is necessary only to discuss the key members of the group, tetracycline and oxytetracycline. These drugs are usually given orally in a dose 250 to 500 mg 6-hourly. They are poorly absorbed and must be given on an empty stomach. Milk and antacids will seriously interfere with their absorption. Their main indications are discussed in the introduction.

Doxycycline and minocycline

These drugs have the advantage of being better absorbed than tetracycline. Doxycycline is long-acting and only has to be given once daily. Both drugs are safer than tetracycline in that they are less likely to produce or worsen renal failure (see below). Their other side effects are the same.

Side effects of tetracyclines

It is probably as well to preface the list of side effects which this drug can cause with the statement that most patients on a short course of treatment rarely experience serious side effects. When tetracycline is given for a long time or in high doses a number of unwanted effects can occur. Some of these are:

1. Anorexia, nausea and vomiting
2. Diarrhoea
3. Monilial or staphylococcal enterocolitis
4. Deterioration of renal function in patients with renal disease (not doxycycline)
5. Deposition in growing teeth and bones.

The anorexia, nausea and vomiting induced by tetracycline in a few patients is not especially noteworthy. Diarrhoea is a side effect in some individuals. This is usually mild and is not often sufficiently severe to warrant stopping treatment. The death of the normal bacterial flora of the bowel which tetracycline induces may cause overgrowth of tetracycline-resistant organisms, notably *Staphylococcus aureus* and monilia throughout the length of the alimentary tract. This complication results in profuse watery diarrhoea and patients may die within 24 hours from dehydration and toxaemia.

Serious deterioration of renal function is due to an antianabolic effect of tetracyclines. These drugs prevent protein synthesis and expose the kidney to increased levels of nitrogenous waste products.

Courses of tetracycline can be damaging to the foetus, after the fourth month of pregnancy and to the the growing child if exhibited when he is less than 12 years old. If the drug *is* given, the deposition in dental enamel may cause malformation and discolouration of the teeth.

Tetracycline should not be administered orally concurrently with oral iron or oral calcium because a complex between antibiotic and element is formed which is non-absorbable. A rare side effect of tetracyclines was acute liver damage which occurred when the drugs were given in large doses intravenously. This extremely serious side effect occurred predominantly when the drugs were used in pregnancy. There are really few indications for giving tetracyclines parenterally and, as stated earlier, patients suffering from common serious infections should receive alternative therapy.

Chloramphenicol

This antibiotic was introduced into clinical practice in 1947. It was at that time obtained from colonies of *Streptomyces venezuelae* but it is now chemically synthesised. Chloramphenicol is a broad spectrum antibiotic with bacteriostatic activity. It may be given orally in a dose of 250 mg four times a day.

This drug is nowadays very seldom used because it may occasionally produce the fatal condition of aplastic anaemia. It is especially likely to do this in children. Aplastic anaemia is a condition where the red cells vanish from the blood very quickly because of marrow failure to produce them. It is a rare side effect of chloramphenicol treatment but you will appreciate that the more patients are given the drug unnecessarily the greater the risk of death from aplastic anaemia for someone who need not have died.

The indications for the drug are infections due to organisms which are resistant to the action of all other antibiotics, typhoid fever and meningitis caused by *Haemophilus influenzae*. Patients with infections due to *Klebsiella pneumoniae* may be treated with chloramphenicol.

THE MACROLIDE GROUP

The important drugs in this group are erythromycin, lincomycin and clindamycin. Lincomycin is now seldom used as it is poorly absorbed and clindamycin is more effective.

Erythromycin has a fairly wide spectrum of antibacterial activity. In serious infections it is less effective than the penicillins or aminoglycosides and its use tends to be confined to treatment of infections of the upper respiratory tract. It penetrates tissue fairly well and this plus its activity against *Staph. aureus* makes it useful for the treatment of middle ear infections and skin diseases. Liver damage was a problem with some of the earlier preparations of this agent but modern drugs are safe. An interesting discovery has been that erythromycin is one of the few drugs which has been shown to be effective in the recently discovered and serious illness known as Legionnaire's disease. It is also of value in the treatment of mycoplasma pneumonia.

Clindamycin

Use of this drug was originally confined to treatment of soft tissue infections involving *Staph. aureas* against which it is particularly effective. This is still the most common indication but recently clindamycin has been found to be effective against anaerobic organisms which colonise the gastrointestinal tract and which tend to be resistant to other forms of therapy. For this reason it is sometimes used in combination with gentamicin in serious systemic infection originating in the abdominal cavity. It is a fairly safe drug but diarrhoea is a common side effect and occasionally a serious form of bowel inflammation known as psuedomembranous colitis may develop during treatment. The usual dose is 150–300 mg 6-hourly.

MISCELLANEOUS DRUGS

Sodium fusidate

This drug has a narrow range of activity but is particularly effective against *Staph. aureas*. It effectively penetrates relatively avascular tissue such as bone, and this makes it a popular choice in combination with other antistaphylococcal agents in the treatment of osteomyelitis. It seems a safe drug but is extremely expensive.

Metronidazole (See also p. 124)

This versatile drug certainly deserves a mention. Originally introduced as therapy for trichimonal infections of the genital tract in women, it has since been shown to be effective in the treatment of a diverse group of conditions including acute ulcerative gingivitis (Vincent's angina) and amoebiasis involving the liver and intestine (see section on imported infections). An important discovery has been its effectiveness in the treatment of infections involving anaerobic organisms originating in the gastrointestinal tract. Metronidazole is used prophylactically to prevent sepsis following abdominal surgery and it is used in combination with a potent broad spectrum antibiotic such as gentamicin should septicaemia develop following surgery. It is a very safe drug which does not seem to cause serious adverse reactions. Nausea, headache and dizziness may occur during therapy but the drug seldom has to be stopped because of this. The dose varies from 4 to 12 200 mg tablets daily, depending on the indication. An intravenous preparation is now available.

ANTITUBERCULOUS AGENTS

Tuberculosis has been one of the great killing diseases of the past two centuries. Despite the advent of effective therapy and a steady decline in the incidence of this condition it remains an important and serious disease even in western communities. The ability of the tubercle bacillus to survive conditions which would kill most other micro-organisms, and the tendency for infection to flair up after lying dormant for many years, single this out as a unique problem which requires a different approach from that adopted for the majority of infectious conditions.

The characteristics of antituberculous therapy are as follows:

1. Treatment must be continued for a long time. Eighteen months to 2 years has been the standard but recent work with new drug regimes has shortened this in some cases to a year or even 9 months
2. It is essential that several drugs are used at once as the tubercle bacillus quickly becomes resistant to single drug therapy. It is usual to commence treatment with three agents then reduce this to two drugs after a few weeks
3. Care must be taken in calculating the exact dose for individual patients. This helps to lessen toxicity which is relatively common with some antituberculous drugs and ensures that the patient is receiving sufficient drug to eradicate infection
4. Careful supervision of the patient to ensure good compliance with the prescribed therapy is essential. If treatment is stopped prematurely infection will recur and the organism may develop resistance to the original drugs. Patients who have recovered from the initial infection are not unnaturally reluctant to continue therapy for many months during which they fell perfectly well. A simple screening test can be performed upon urine samples to check that they are indeed taking the drug.

In this section only 'the first line' antituberculous drugs in common use will be discussed. Use of the less well-known drugs in cases resistant to conventional therapy is a specialised topic outside the scope of this book.

Streptomycin

This drug has already been discussed in the section on aminoglycoside antibiotics. It remains one of the most effective antituberculous drugs available and is still included in many drug regimes. It has to be given by injection and this fact plus its toxicity are major drawbacks. For this reason, treatment schedules have been developed in the last few years which substitute rifampicin for streptomycin. The results have been equally good. Originally streptomycin was combined with sodium aminosalicylate and isoniazid. This combination is still used occasionally but streptomycin, isioniazid and ethambutol is now more popular. The usual dose is 0.75 to 1.0 mg per day, given intramuscularly.

Isoniazid

This chemotherapeutic agent is still an important part of all modern regimes for the treatment of TB. It is a very effective drug which produces little serious toxicity. Occasionally hepatitis, peripheral neutitis or inflammation of the optic nerve may develop. An interesting finding has been that approximately half the population (this proportion varies from country to country) are slow inactivators of isoniazid. This means that their livers contain reduced quantities of the enzyme necessary for breakdown of the drug. This tendency to be a slow inactivator is an inherited one and these individuals naturally tend to accumulate the drug in their body with the resulting increase in side effects. This fact should be borne in mind if a patient develops side effects while receiving isoniazid. Peripheral neuritis and visual upsets respond to treatment with pyridoxine (vitamin B6) and this is often administered along with the drug. The average adult dose of isoniazid is 200-400 mg daily.

Sodium aminosalicylate

This was an essential part of the original antituberculous drug schedules but because of the frequency of side effects and the advent of more effective drugs it is now seldom used. Large doses (10 to 20 g daily) are necessary and patients find these difficult to swallow. The taste is unpleasant and nausea is very common.

Ethambutol

This is an effective antituberculous drug which is now used instead of sodium aminosalicylate. As with all the antituberculous drugs it must be used in combination with other agents (usually streptomycin and isoniazid). A serious side effect of treatment is inflammation of the optic nerve, with resulting blindness. This seems to be commoner when high doses of the drug are used and fortunately recovers following withdrawal of the drug in most cases. Any visual disturbance in a patient receiving ethambutol must be treated very seriously. The dose of ethambutol varies according to the patient's weight.

Rifampicin

This is a newer drug which is particularly effective in the treatment of tuberculosis. Indeed it is quite likely that the combination of isoniazid, ethambutol and rifampicin will become the most popular 'first line' treatment for new cases. The main hazard of this drug is its tendency to produce liver damage and liver function tests should be checked periodically during therapy. Rifampicin also speeds up the breakdown of other drugs in the liver and this may render the contraceptive pill ineffective, with predictable results. Rifampicin has an unusual effect in that it turns the sputum and urine of patients a reddish colour and they should be warned of this. The dose varies according to body weight.

ANTIFUNGAL ANTIBIOTICS

A few antibiotics act principally against fungi. The ones used most commonly are nystatin, amphotericin B and griseofulvin.

Nystatin

This is one of the most widely used antifungal agents. It is effective against *Candida albicans* which is a common infectious agent causing oral and occasionally anal and vaginal thrush. It is an alternative to the older treatment with gentian violet which although effective is very unsightly. Nystatin is not absorbed from the gastrointestinal tract and must be applied locally to infections of the skin, pharynx and genital area. It is customary to give 100000 units (1 ml suspension) 6-hourly in oral candidiasis but in many cases larger doses up to 500000 units 6-hourly may be more effective. It is important to remember that the drug is acting locally and the longer the time it is in contact with the infected surface the better. For this reason, lozenges may be preferable.

Amphotericin B

This is the most potent antifungal agent available. Used in the form of lozenges it is very effective for the treatment of oral candidiasis and it is not absorbed by this route. For the treatment of serious systemic fungal infections which can develop in patients with impaired immunity, amphotericin is administered intravenously. The main limitation to therapy is toxicity in the form of renal damage which is almost invariable when this drug is used. A careful watch must be kept on the renal function during therapy. A modest rise in the creatinine levels in the blood is allowable and in many cases the damage is reversible. Severe irreversible renal damage may, however, occur, if use of the drug is prolonged. This is regarded as an acceptable hazard as amphotericin is the only really effective agent available for treating systemic fungal infections which will otherwise prove fatal.

Fluocytosine

This drug can be given orally or parenterally for treatment of systemic fungal infections. It can also be used in conjunction with amphotericin. When used alone it is not as effective for treatment of severe infections but is safer. Marrow depression and liver damage are the main hazards.

Imidazoles

This is a new group of drugs currently under development which are effective against a wide range of fungi. The drug best known in this country is clotrimazole (Canestan) which is only available for topical treatment of topical infections of the skin and genitalia. It is probably more effective than nystatin and certainly has a much wider range of activity against different fungi. It is certain that new agents in this group will be available in the future for parenteral administration in serious fungal infections.

Griseofulvin

This is an unusual antifungal drug which is only effective against tinea (ringworm) infections. It is therefore of no value in the treatment of candidiasis. Griseofulvin is administered orally and is concentrated in keratin making it effective treatment for fungal infections of the hair and nails. The rule to remember about griseofulvin is that it works best on infections at the top of the body and less well as one proceeds downwards. Thus infections of the scalp respond quickly and satisfactorily to griseofulvin, fingernail infections may take 6 months to improve while toenail infections may require treatment for as long as a year. The dose is 0.5 to 1 g per day taken by mouth in one dose. A useful tip to give your patient is that griseofulvin is best absorbed after a fatty meal. Side effects are rare.

THE COLLECTION OF SPECIMENS FOR THE BACTERIOLOGIST

Rational and effective antibiotic or chemotherapeutic treatment demands that the organism being treated be sensitive to the action of the agent being used. It is therefore necessary in many cases (and absolutely vital, in some) that the doctor have a clear idea of the sensitivity of the offending organism so that he may choose the appropriate antibiotic. It is standard practice to take a sample of the infected material whether it be sputum, cerebrospinal fluid, or pus from a draining wound, and send it to the bacteriological laboratory. The bacteriologist then lays some of the sample on a series of culture plates and allows the organisms to grow undisturbed on these plates over a 24 hour period. Each plate contains a different antibiotic. Bacteria which are resistant to the action of an antibiotic grow happily in its presence. Bacteria which are sensitive to the antibiotic will fail to grow. It is therefore possible to tell, merely by glancing at the culture plates, the sensitivity and resistance of an organism.

The part which you play in all this is an important one. You will often be responsible for collecting the sample of the infected material which is to be sent to the laboratory. Always try to ensure that only the sample and nothing else enters the sterile tube or container which is supplied by the bacteriologist. It is sometimes difficult to know whether a certain organism is responsible for an infection or is merely a contaminant from the skin of the patient's body or the nurse's fingers. Always try to make the interval between the collection of the sample for culture and its arrival in the laboratory as short as possible. The organisms in infected material may die if they are left in a container which stands on the ward desk for a number of hours. The bacteriologist will then fail to culture the organisms and their antibiotic sensitivity will remain unknown. If a few hours' delay is unavoidable try to avoid subjecting the sample to extremes of heat or cold. The best place to keep material which is to be submitted for bacteriological examination is in an oven kept at body temperature.

By attention to details such as these you will increase your patient's chances of a rapid recovery. Carelessness in the collection of samples for the bacteriologist cannot be too strongly condemned for utlimately it is you patient, not you, who may have to pay the cost of this.

DRUGS USED IN THE TREATMENT OF COMMON INFESTATIONS AND IMPORTED DISEASES

Tropical diseases and infestation with worms of one kind or another constitute a major scourge of mankind. There are today many immigrants who come into temperate zones carrying communicable diseases from the tropics with them. Air travel is rendering distances between countries relatively smaller. We live, in fact, in a contracting world. A major medical consequence of this is the increasing amount of tropical medicine seen in temperate zones.

This chapter describes the drugs which are used in the treatment of some of the diseases more commonly encountered in the tropics. The treatment of worms found in tropical and non-tropical zones is also discussed.

MALARIA

Malaria is the most important infectious disease imported into this country. There has been a marked increase in its incidence in the last few years mainly due to increased air travel. It is possible, therefore, and indeed quite likely, that you will come across cases while nursing in general medical wards. It is important that this condition is recognised quickly and effective treatment started.

In order to grasp the principles which underlie the rational treatment of malaria, you must first understand the way in which the disease enteres the body, how it lives in the body and how it causes its effect on the body.

Malaria is usually transmitted to a healthy individual following the bite of an infected mosquito. The mosquito itself becomes infected as a result of having bitten a subject with malarial parasites circulating in his blood stream. When the mosquito bites it both sucks up blood from the individual and leaves some of its own secretions behind in that individual's blood stream. The sequence then is that an initially healthy mosquito, usually an anopheline female mosquito (*Anophelus* is a certain genus of mosquito) bites an infected individual, receives some of his malarial parasites and later transmits them to another individual by biting. Once the malarial parasites which cause the disease have entered the blood stream they make for the liver where they bread and multiply. At a certain critical stage when they have multiplied many times they invade the blood stream. To do this they leave the liver and enter the red cells in the blood stream. Once in the red cells the parasites breed still further and multiply. After an interval varying from 24 to 72 hours they burst out of the infected red cell and each parasite then invades another cell and so the process goes on.

The various stages of parasite development in the mosquito, the liver and the blood are given names such as the sporozoite stage, merozoite stage, trophozoite stage. It is not necessary for you to know about this because these terms can be confusing and tend to complicate the picture. What you should realise, however, is that most of the drugs given to patients with malaria cannot reach the parasites and destroy them once they are hiding in the liver. These patients require special treatment to effect a *radical cure.*

Treatment of malaria can be thought of under three headings.

1. Drugs given to suppress the occurrence of malaria in a person living in or passing through a malarial area who is exposed to the bites of infected mosquitoes. (Prophylaxis)
2. Drugs given to kill malarial parasites once they have invaded the blood stream from the liver and are multiplying in large numbers within the red cells. (Treatment of an acute attack of overt malaria)
3. Drugs given as special treatment to effect a radical cure of malaria parasites hidden in the liver. (Radical cure.)

Drugs used in suppression of malaria (prophylaxis)

The idea here is to kill the malarial parasites appearing in the blood stream as soon as they start to leave the liver before they have a chance to multiply in the red blood cells. There are four main drugs any one of which may be used to do this.

1. Chloroquine phosphate
2. Amodiaquine hydrochloride
3. Pyrimethamine
4. Proguanil hydrochloride

Because these drugs are being used to prevent a relatively few parasites from the liver gaining a foothold in the blood stream rather than to kill a very large number of parasites which have had a chance to multiply in the blood stream, a small dose of each of them is sufficient. The first three drugs mentioned above have the great advantage that suppression is achieved by taking them only once a week. Proguanil, however, must be taken daily. Pyrimethamine and proguanil act not only on parasites as they leave the liver and start to enter the blood stream but they also kill most kinds of malarial parasites as soon as they first enter the liver before they have had a chance to breed and hide themselves in that organ. These drugs, however, do not have this action on *Plasmodium vivax* infections. This malarial parasite requires special treatment to eradicate it from the liver.

Treatment of an overt malarial attack

In an overt clinical attack of malaria, due to a very large number of parasites in the blood, the patient has periods of severe rigors with high pyrexia alternating with periods of drenching sweats. Overt attacks of malaria are treated either by:

1. Chloroquine phosphate   *or*
2. Amodiaquine hydrochloride.

These drugs are used in higher dosage than is required for suppressive treatment. A typical dose of chloroquine phosphate is 600 mg followed 6 hours later by 300 mg. A further two doses of 300 mg are then given at 24 hour intervals. Toxic effects with chloroquine are rare in the treatment of malaria. If the drug is used in very high doses to treat patients with rheumatoid arthritis serious side effects do occur.

In the emergency treatment of acute fulminating forms of malaria caused by the *Plasmodium falciparum* parasite, chloroquine is administered intramuscularly. Another drug sometimes used to treat this condition is quinine. This is given by slow intravenous infusion. Although quinine is of historical interest (it was the drug first used in the treatment of malaria) it is now seldom used to treat other forms of malaria because of potentially dangerous side effects.

Radical cure of malaria

As has been mentioned above, none of the drugs used to kill malarial parasites in the blood or most parasites at an early stage of development in the liver, act on infections established in the liver. For this reason these infections used to be extremely difficult to eradicate. No matter which drug was given or the dosage that was used, the parasite sheltered safely in the liver and would re-emerge into the blood to cause clinical recrudescences of malaria for some years after the initial infection had been 'treated'. Recently, the situation has improved. The advent of drugs of the 8-aminoquinoline family has provided an effective means of killing the parasite even when it is in the liver.

The most commonly used of the 8-aminoquinilones and the drug of this family least toxic to the patient, is primaquine phosphate. This is given in a daily dose of 15 mg for a fortnight. One course of treatment is usually quite effective. The patient is thus released from the threat of an acute attack of malaria.

Primaquine has an interesting side effect. When it is given to genetically susceptible individuals it causes the development of acute haemolytic anaemia. The susceptibility to develop acute haemolysis after being given primaquine is a trait that the patient inherits. Curiously enough this very trait seems to be associated with increased natural resistance to malarial parasites. Most people with this trait do not, in fact, need to be treated with primaquine.

Proguanil interferes with the metabolism of primaquine and leads to the development of very high levels of this drug in the blood. There is then a danger of primaquine-induced jaundice because this drug has a toxic effect on the liver cells in high concentration.

Parasite resistance to antimalarial drugs

A problem which is of current importance is how to deal with the increasing numbers of malarial parasites acquiring resistance to chloroquine. There is no easy answer to this question except to treat all malarial infections adequately and to change immediately to a different drug as soon as drug resistance in the parasite is suspected. At the present, resistant infections are usually treated with quinine despite its toxicity. The search for new antimalarial drugs is being vigorously pursued.

DRUGS USED IN THE TREATMENT OF LEPROSY

Leprosy, a chronic mutilating disease of the skin and peripheral nerves is caused by an acid-alcohol fast bacillus which is in many ways similar to the tubercle bacillus. The leprosy bacillus is amenable to treatment by a number of different agents. For drug treatment of leprosy to be effective, it must be given in many cases for a number of years. The most important drugs used to treat patients with leprosy are as follows:

1. Dapsone
2. Clofazimine
3. Rifampicin.

Dapsone

Dapsone, the most generally useful drug against leprosy, is given orally beginning with small doses (25 to 100 mg twice weekly). These are slowly increased until the patient is receiving 300 to 400 mg twice weekly. Dapsone is an effective antileprotic agent but treatment must be continued for months or even, in some cases, years. The emergence of drug resistant strains is now on the increase.

Side effects of dapsone

These may be severe and therefore caution is required when the dose of the drug is being increased. A generalised flare up of the disease may occur in the early months of treatment. This is known as a 'lepra reaction'. There may be increased pain experienced by the patient due to swelling of the peripheral nerves.

Skin rashes, in particular an erythema nodosum-like picture, may occur and anaemia is also seen. If any of these conditions appear this is a clear indication for stopping treatment with dapsone. Should the side effects persist it may be necessary to give corticosteroid drugs to control them.

Clofazimine

The most recent of the drugs used to treat patients with leprosy, clofazimine appears to be one of the best. The drug is given orally in daily doses ranging from 100 to 600 mg. Clofazimine is effective in patients who are resistant to the action of dapsone. The drug is a red dye and is deposited in the skin, in body fat and in lymph nodes. The resultant pinkish discoloration has limited its use in patients with light pigmentation (particularly in the Chinese) but not in darker coloured patients.

Lepra reactions are encountered less frequently during treatment with clofazimine than with dapsone and this is to be counted another advantage of the drug.

Rifampicin

This antibiotic which has already been mentioned in the treatment of tuberculosis is very effective for the treatment of leprosy. Unfortunately it is also very expensive and this limits its use in the developing countries.

DRUGS USED IN THE TREATMENT OF AMOEBIASIS

Patients who harbour the *Entamoeba histolytica,* the parasite which causes amoebiasis, may have either acute dysentery, chronic dysentery or amoebic hepatitis.

Treatment of acute amoebic dysentery

This is an important condition as it is quite common and can be mistaken for ulcerative colitis. This is an important distinction as the usual treatment for ulcerative colitis is corticosteroids and this can be dangerous in a patient suffering from amoebic dysentery.

The best drug in the treatment of patients suffering from acute dysentery caused by infestation with the *Entamoeba histolytica* is metronidazole.

Metronidazole

This drug has already been discussed earlier in the chapter. One of its important indications is the treatment of amoebiasis. It is now the treatment of choice for acute amoebic infections of the bowel and liver and is also very effective in the eradication of amoebic cysts from asymptomatic carriers. As stated earlier, it is relatively non-toxic and for treatment of amoebiasis is usually given in a dose of 400 mg thrice daily for 5 days.

Emetine hydrochloride

Emetine is effective in treatment of tissue infections by amoebae but will not eradicate the protozoa from the intestine. It is given by intramuscular injection. It is a dangerous drug in overdosage and patients should never receive more than 60 mg per day. The requirements of a patient for emetine are usually expressed in terms of his body weight (1 mg of emetine being given for every kg of patient). A course of the drug should not exceed 5 days. If these precautions are observed you are unlikely to encounter side effects in your patients being treated with emetine. It is a wise step nonetheless to check the blood pressure twice daily because hypotension is a feature of overdosage with this drug.

ENTERIC FEVERS

Typhoid and paratyphoid occur quite commonly in this country. Immigrants and holidaymakers being the usual sufferers. Cloramphenicol has been the drug of choice for a long time but some strains of salmonella resistant to this drug have developed. A number of other drugs are suitable for treatment, including ampicillin, amoxycillin and cotrimoxazole. All of these drugs have already been discussed earlier in this chapter. Whatever drug is used, treatment must be continued for at least 2 weeks and the doses of drugs used tend to be higher than for their usual indications.

ANTHELMINTHICS

Anthelminthics are drugs which are used in the treatment of patients who are infested with worms. There is a large variety of worms many of which are found exclusively in tropical climates while others occur both in tropical and temperate zones. The commoner varieties of worms which afflict mankind are schistosomes, filaria, tapeworms, threadworms, roundworms and hookworms.

DRUGS USED IN THE TREATMENT OF PATIENTS WITH SCHISTOSOMIASIS

Schistosomes are found in infested ditches, canals and lakes. They enter human beings who bathe in infected water by penetrating the skin and so gain access to the blood stream. These parasites are then carried either to the liver or the bladder or the lungs and in these sites they cause the damage which is responsible for the clinical symptoms of schistosomiasis. In the past, antimony compounds were the drugs of choice in schistosomiasis. They are toxic drugs, however, and niridazole is now the most popular agent.

Niridazole

This agent is effective in all forms of schistosomiasis. It can be given orally for a course of treatment of 10 days. The drug can cause unwanted effects on the brain including confusional states and epilepsy. Some patients notice that the urine becomes discoloured while they are receiving niridazole. A typical adult dose is 0.8 g twice daily.

Antimony sodium tartrate

This drug commonly causes nausea and vomiting after administration. If large doses are given too quickly myocardial damage may occur. Antimony sodium tartrate is given by intravenous injection beginning with doses of the order of 30 mg thrice weekly and increasing to doses of 120 mg thrice weekly.

The patient is usually given the injection when he is fasting because of the liability of the drug to induce nausea and vomiting. It is also common practice for the patient to lie down while the drug is being administered. If any of the injection leaks outside the vein a severe reaction manifested by local tissue necrosis is liable to occur. A course of treatment entails giving an adult patient about 2 g of the drug.

Stibophen

This drug is less effective than antimony sodium tartrate in achieving a permanent cure of schistosomiasis. It has the advantage of being less toxic, however, and it can be given by intramuscular injection. As with antimony sodium tartrate, the course of treatment begins with small doses of the drug which are increased to a maximum of 5 ml (300 mg of stibophen) every two days.

A course of treatment consists of 40 to 75 ml.

Sodium antimonylgluconate

This is an alternative preparation to antimony sodium tartrate. It is given by intravenous injection in a dose of 190 mg for six days.

Stibocaptate

This drug is given intramuscularly. The dose is 500 mg given daily for five days.

Lucanthone

Lucanthone is given by mouth. It is most active against schistosomal infections of the urinary tract. Side effects are frequently encountered in patients receiving treatment with lucanthone and include nausea and vomiting, epigastric and abdominal pain, headache, dizziness and mental depression. The dose is 1 g given twice daily for three days.

DRUGS USED IN THE TREATMENT OF PATIENTS WITH FILARIASIS

Filarial worms are found in the lymphatic system where they

produce blockage to the free drainage of lymph. In chronic infections this may lead to the condition known as elephantiasis.

Diethylcarbamazine

Diethylcarbamazine is the drug most commonly used. This drug produces effective destruction of all kinds of young filarial worms but is less active against some adult worms. Some forms of adult worms are killed by this agent, however, while others are rendered incapable of breeding.

It is usual to start treatment with diethylcarbamazine in a small dose (usually 2 to 6 mg per kg body weight per day). The reason for using a small dose initially is that the destruction of the young filarial worms produced by this agent is liable to trigger off an allergic reaction to the dead worms. This reaction is manifested by fever, itchiness of the skin and joint pains. If the eye has been invaded by worms, as is sometimes the case, a flare of the disease will occur in the eye. In many patients much larger doses may be required for 3 to 4 weeks to control the disease. When an initial small dose has been tolerated for a week or so, the amount of the drug given to the patient is cautiously increased to levels of 24 to 49 mg per kg body weight per day.

Diethylcarbamazine is the drug of choice for filariasis.

DRUGS USED IN THE TREATMENT OF PATIENTS WITH TAPEWORMS

Tapeworms are intestinal parasites acquired by consuming infected meat or fish which has been imperfectly cooked. These worms are found both in temperate and in tropical climes. *Taenia saginata*, the tapeworm acquired after eating contaminated beef is the one most commonly found in Britain. *Taenia solium* occurs in infested pork and is destroyed only when pork is properly cooked. It is a wise precaution to ensure that all kinds of pigmeat and beef which you eat have been cooked right through.

The principle behind the successful treatment of a patient with a tapeworm is to give a drug which causes the worm to relax its hold upon the wall of the intestine and then to flush it out of the bowel by means of a purgative. The drugs commonly used to do this are dichlorophen and niclosamide.

Dichlorophen

Before dichlorophen, a purgative (usually magnesium sulphate), is given to clear the bowel of food which might protect the worm. After treatment the worm is expelled in a partially digested state and it is not possible to find the head. The stools should, however, be examined 2 to 3 months after treatment with dichlorophen to ensure that tapeworm segments are no longer present.

The dose of the drug is 70 mg per kg body weight given in divided doses over the period of one day.

Niclosamide

Like dichlorophen this drug has a direct toxic action on tapeworms. It is not absorbed to any extent from the intestine and side effects are rare.

DRUGS USED IN THE TREATMENT OF PATIENTS WITH THREADWORMS

Infestation of the lumen of the rectum and anal canal with threadworms occurs very commonly in young children. These worms emerge at night from the anus and deposit their eggs on the perianal skin. This causes intense pruritus and sleeplessness. Threadworms can be detected by a doctor (or by a nurse who knows how to use a microscope) by rubbing a piece of cellophane firmly over the perianal skin. The cellophane is then placed on a slide and examined under the microscope for the eggs of the female threadworm. Remember that if one person in a family is affected it is likely that all of the family is affected and will require treatment.

Piperazine is effective against threadworms.

Piperazine

This drug may be given in tablet form (as piperazine adipate or citrate) or in the form of an elixir or syrup (piperazine citrate). The dose varies with the age of the patient. The syrup is pleasant tasting and it is thus often more easily administered to young children than tablets. The dose for children less than 2 years of age is 2.5 ml per day; 3 to 5 years of age, 2.5 ml thrice daily, 6 to 12 years of age, 5 ml twice daily and 13 years or more, 5 ml thrice daily. A course of treatment is usually given for 1 week and this is repeated after an interval of 1 week to prevent reinfestation.

Viprynium

This is given as a liquid in a dose of 5 mg per kg body weight. Usually a single dose suffices to eradicate threadworms but it is often worthwhile giving a second dose 2 weeks after the first to prevent reinfestation by threadworm eggs swallowed before the first treatment was given. This drug causes the stools to become red and it may cause staining of the clothes. It is necessary to mention this to parents whose children are being treated with viprynium.

DRUGS USED IN THE TREATMENT OF PATIENTS WITH ROUNDWORMS

Roundworms may occur in large numbers in the small intestine of many subjects living in tropical areas. These worms can sometimes cause intestinal obstruction.

Piperazine is effective in the treatment of roundworms. The worms are paralysed and release their hold on the lumen of the bowel. They are then passed in the stool. In children with heavy infestations the regimen of treatment with piperazine is similar to that used in the treatment of threadworms.

Bephenium

This drug is active against roundworms. The dose employed is that used in the treatment of hookworm infestation, namely 5 g (see below).

Thiabendazole

This is a relatively new agent for the treatment of roundworms but it is also active against a variety of other types of worms.

DRUGS USED IN THE TREATMENT OF PATIENTS WITH HOOKWORMS

Hookworms, which occur in tropical countries, fix themselves to the wall of the small bowel and may cause heavy loss of blood which leads to iron deficiency anaemia. Bephenium and tetrachlorethylene are active against hookworms.

Bephenium

This drug is less toxic than tetrachlorethylene because it is very poorly absorbed from the bowel. Purging is not required when bephenium is administered and like tetrachlorethylene (see below) a single dose is often effective. Multiple doses are occasionally required to eradicate all of the worms in a heavily infested patient. The dose of bephenium is 5 g suspended in a glass of water given to your patient after an overnight fast.

Tetrachlorethylene

Your patient should fast overnight and be given a bulk purgative in the morning. Castor oil should not be employed as this aids absorption of tetrachlorethylene. The drug is then given in a dose of 3 ml. Two hours later another purgative is given to effect the removal of the worms and the tetrachlorethylene from the lumen of the bowel. This drug is more toxic than bephenium but because it is cheaper it is used a lot in poorer countries.

6

Drugs used in disorders of the central nervous system

HYPNOTICS

Many patients cannot sleep in a hospital ward at night. Worry about their medical problems, anxiety about whether they are going to get better, pain or general discomfort, all of these things make it difficult to sleep. The problem is compounded by noise from other patients (and dare it be said from the nursing and medical staff). There is a real need for the use of hypnotics to induce sleep in these circumstances.

Outside of hospital however there are many more patients who take hypnotics than have real need of them. Withdrawal of hypnotics once started may cause temporary insomnia and it is possibly for this reason that these drugs are difficult to stop. You can help here by explaining to your patient before his discharge from hospital that he may have one or two sleepless nights at home initially but that this will soon cease in a few days of its own accord. Reassurance of this sort may prevent him from asking his general practitioner for more sleeping tablets.

In some patients difficulty in sleeping may be the first sign of endogenous depression particularly if the patient wakens at 4 or 5 a.m. and cannot get back to sleep. Treatment here may be anti-depressant therapy and not by hypnotics.

The most commonly used hypnotic agents currently are members of a class of compounds known as the benzodiazepines. These agents also have tranquillising properties. The drug most widely used in this class as a hypnotic is nitrazepam.

Benzodiazepines

This group of sedative drugs was introduced in the 1960s and its members are amongst the most commonly used drugs both inside and outside hospital. The main reason for their popularity is their extreme safety both for day to day use and also when they are taken in overdose. Fatality resulting from overdose of a benzodiazepine drug is extremely rare although of course the danger is greater when the drug is taken in combination with another drug such as barbiturates or alcohol. Although benzodiazepine drugs are very safe in the majority of patients it should be remembered that this does not hold true for individuals with serious respiratory or hepatic disease who may become comatose after a normally safe dose of any sedative drug.

Nitrazepam

This is the most commonly used hypnotic drug in hospital. It is rapid in its onset of action and lasts for approximately 8 hours. Patients waken feeling refreshed rather than muddled. The drug therefore contrasts very well with barbiturates which are very dangerous when taken in overdosage and are apt to leave patients rather muddled and confused. This is especially so in the elderly.

Rather than by producing a state of heavy sedation nitrazepam acts as a hypnotic by relieving the anxieties which occupy a patient's mind, keeping him or her awake. This holds true for the other benzodiazepine drugs mentioned in this section.

Diazepam

You may be surprised to see diazepam appear in a section on hypnotics as it is generally used as a tranquilliser. However as noted above a state of tranquillity will lead to sleep and diazepam is as effective and safe in this respect as nitrazepam. It is, incidentally, cheaper. The usual hypnotic dose is 5 to 10 mg at night.

Flurazepam

This is a newer drug which is generally used as a hypnotic. It has no real advantages over nitrazepam or diazepam and is more expensive. The usual dose is 15 to 30 mg per day.

Although only three of the most commonly used benzodiazepines have been mentioned in this section any other members of the group, which includes chlordiazepoxide, oxazepam, lorazepam and medazepam, may be used as hypnotic. As a general rule it is wise to use only one or two drugs routinely and to know them well.

Barbiturates

These drugs are narcotics with sedative and hypnotic actions in therapeutic dosage. They form a large class of compounds all of which are synthesised from a parent substance, barbituric acid. Barbiturates can be classified into drugs with a long duration of action (such as phenobarbitone), drugs with a medium duration of action (such as amylobarbitone) and drugs with a very brief duration of action (such as thiopentone). Barbiturates are usually given orally but can be given parenterally. Thiopentone is given by intravenous injection and is used as an anaesthetic agent.

Action of the barbiturates

These drugs are powerful cerebral depressants. In small doses they depress the cerebral cortex to a slight degree and act as sedatives taking the edge off patients' anxieties and fears. In larger doses barbiturates have a hypnotic action for they depress the cerebral cortex effectively and to such an extent that first drowsiness, then sleep supervenes. In overdosage these drugs induce depression not only of the higher cortical centres but also of the vital centres (such as the respiratory centre) in the medulla. Death from overdosage of barbiturates is usually caused by the effects of these drugs on the respiratory centre.

A point worth knowing about the barbiturates is that they potentiate the action of alcohol and other cerebral depressants. You must always make sure that your patients realise that they should not drink alcohol while they are taking these drugs.

Barbiturates are excreted in the urine and by the liver in the bile. For this reason, patients with impaired renal and hepatic function should be given barbiturates with extreme caution.

Uses of barbiturates

These drugs have four main uses in clinical practice:

1. They combat anxiety
2. They induce sleep
3. They control epileptic attacks and lessen their frequency
4. They are used to induce anaesthesia.

Treatment of anxiety with barbiturates

The barbiturate which is traditionally used to treat anxiety is phenobarbitone. It is given in small doses of the order of 30 mg two or three times a day. In contrast to most other members of the barbiturate family, phenobarbitone is not an effective hypnotic. The drug has a duration of action of roughly 12 to 24 hours and doses required to induce sleep are usually quite large. For both of these reasons patients given phenobarbitone in hypnotic doses often feel muzzy-headed the following day. There is little doubt that barbiturates are still overprescribed for the treatment of anxiety. They have been completely superceded in the treatment of this condition by the benzodiazepines. Often anxiety may co-exist with depression and barbiturates may merely worsen the depression and then provide the patient with a way of committing suicide.

Barbiturates as hypnotics

Barbiturates with a medium duration of action have been the first-choice hypnotic agents for some years but have now been supplanted by nitrazepam for reasons described above. It must be stressed that there is now no reason for using barbiturates as hypnotics in new patients. Many patients, however, have been using the drugs for many years and although an attempt should be made to switch them to a safer alternative this often fails. You will therefore continue to see these drugs prescribed but much less frequently than in the past.

There is a large number of these drugs and there is not much to choose between any of them. Their duration of action ranges from 3 to 8 hours depending on the drug used and the individual response of a particular patient. The names of the most commonly used barbiturates in this class are: butobarbitone; amylobarbitone; pentobarbitone; quinalbarbitone; cyclobarbitone.

Elderly patients should never be given barbiturates. These drugs frequently induce confusion and disorientation in the aged so that they tend to forget where they are. Many old people tend to sleep short hours and it is common practice for some of them when they are at home to get up at 3 or 4 in the morning to make themselves a cup of tea. Insistence on continuous sleep from 10 o'clock at night till 7 o'clock is unrealistic, and thoughtful reassurance perhaps reinforced by a cup of tea is much preferred to heavy sedation.

Barbiturates as anaesthetics

The short-acting barbiturates are used to induce anaesthesia. The best known and the most frequently used of these is the drug thiopentone. Because thiopentone is extremely irritant it is given slowly by intravenous injection, great care being taken to avoid extravasation of the drug into the subcutaneous tissues where it produces tissue sloughing and necrosis. The effect of thiopentone in causing unconsciousness is apparent almost immediately following the beginning of the injection. The action of the drug lasts for approximately 20 minutes and therefore it is not suitable for maintaining anaesthesia throughout the operation.

There is some evidence that barbiturates lower the pain theshold. Patients who have received thiopentone often require fairly large doses of analgesics postoperatively to control their pain.

Laryngeal spasm sometimes occurs following the induction of anaesthesia with thiopentone. For this reason the drug should be administered only by an experienced anaesthetist who has facilities to carry out laryngeal intubation.

Side effects of barbiturates

The main problems associated with the use of barbiturates are excessive sedation, the extreme effects when taken in overdose and the possibility of drug dependence developing. True adverse effects such as nausea, vomiting and drug-induced rashes do occur but are relatively uncommon. An interesting side effect of the barbiturates is their ability to increase the activity of certain specialised enzymes within the liver. This effect is known as enzyme induction. This may be important if another drug is being administered at the same time which is extensively metabolised in the liver. A good example is warfarin. When a patient is anticoagulated with warfarin and barbiturates are started, warfarin is broken down more quickly and a larger dose is then needed to maintain the previous anticoagulated state. It is thought that barbiturates occasionally result in increased breakdown of activated folic acid. This probably only occurs in patients who have a relatively poor diet. When folic acid deficiency develops then megaloblastic anaemia results. Barbiturates may also induce the breakdown of vitamin D, resulting in osteomalacia or rickets in children.

OTHER HYPNOTICS

Chloral hydrate

This is a safe, mild hypnotic which is especially valuable in children and young infants. It has unfortunately a very bitter taste and leaves an unpleasant aftertaste in the mouth. Attempts to disguise this taste with orange juice or peppermint water do not always meet with success and many a dose of this drug has ended its life by being spat on to the floor. In order to overcome these difficulties a derivative closely allied to chloral hydrate which can be given in tablet form is often preferred. This is dichloralphenazone ('Welldorm'). Triclofos is another derivative of value.

Glutethimide

This drug induces sleep lasting for approximately 6 hours. It is occasionally used. Although fairly safe when used in normal doses, glutethimide is very dangerous in overdose. Its routine use therefore is not recommended and the benzodiazepines which are every bit as effective and much safer are preferred.

Mandrax

This consists of a hypnotic drug (methaqualone) and an antihistamine with sedative properties (diphenhydramine) in a power-fully hypnotic mixture with a rapid onset of action. Mandrax is no longer used routinely as it is very dangerous when taken in overdose. It has also been subject to abuse and is occasionally used by drug addicts.

Promethazine

Most of the antihistamine group have some sedative action and promethazine, one of the most commonly used drugs, is still occasionally employed as a hypnotic. It is a long-acting drug with only mild effects. It is relatively safe but has no advantages over nitrazepam.

Paraldehyde

You may still see paraldehyde being used occasionally but it is really of historical interest only. It is a relatively safe hypnotic and can be effective when given intramuscularly in the treatment of status epilepticus. It is, however, a disagreeable drug both for the patient and the nurse. It has a most unpleasant odour and as it is partly excreted in the breath, patients who have received an injection of paraldehyde reek of it for some hours. It is perhaps not sufficiently well known that the patient is able to smell the paraldehyde as he excretes it via the lungs. If paraldehyde is being used it should be drawn up into the syringe and injected very soon afterwards as it has a tendency to dissolve plastic.

TRANQUILLISERS

There are two main groups of tranquillising drugs. The first group comprises those drugs which are used to relieve the symptoms of anxiety. The benzodiazepines, and to a much lesser extent, the barbiturates form this group, and as stated earlier these drugs are also used as hypnotics. This group is known as the minor tran-quillisers. The second group consists of those drugs which are used to combat extreme agitation in the very disturbed patient who is usually suffering from severe mental illness. The pheno-thiazines are the most important members of this group which is known as the major tranquillisers.

MINOR TRANQUILLISERS

These are drugs which produce changes in the emotional tone of the patient so as to relieve anxiety and mental tension. It is unclear whether there is more anxiety and mental tension around today than previously, or whether it is merely that the offer of drugs which powerfully release the unquiet mind from its worries is gratefully seized on by those for whom previously there was little effective remedy other than addiction to opium or alcohol. Whatever the reason, tranquillisers are one of the most commonly consumed drugs of those that are issued on prescription. They probably rank second to purgatives in frequency of use and it may be that in the majority of cases there is as little real justification for the use of the one as there is for the use of the other.

All of these agents may induce drowsiness particularly if the patient consumes alcohol with which they interact. You should warn your patient about this.

Benzodiazepines

This group is comprised of a fairly large number of drugs including diazepam, chlordiazepoxide, oxazepam, lorazepam and medazepam. As mentioned earlier, two other benzodiazepines, nitrazepam and flurazepam are usually used as hypnotics although their effects are really very similar to the other members of this family of drugs. Diazepam and chlordiazepoxide are the two drugs most commonly prescribed and we will confine our discussion to them. Diazepam is usually prescribed in a dose of 2 to 5 mg three times daily, and chlordiazepoxide 5 to 10 mg three times daily. Both are very safe but will tend to produce drowsiness in excessive doses. Elderly people are especially at risk and may also develop ataxia (unsteadiness of gait). Other side effects such as nausea and drug rashes are uncommon with the benzodiazepine group as a whole.

Given intravenously diazepam or chlordiazepoxide are each enormously successful in sedating the unruly or aggressive individual. They are very useful drugs for the control of status epilepticus and are particularly valuable in the sedation of patients in delirium tremens.

Barbiturates

The barbiturate drugs are still used to treat symptoms of anxiety, but as stated in the section on hypnotics their continued use in this situation cannot be recommended. They are discussed in more detail on pages 133–136.

MAJOR TRANQUILLISERS

These are drugs which are administered in order to control the seriously disturbed patient. The situations in which these drugs are used vary from the young schizophrenic or manic patient to the elderly confused individual whose noisy agitation can easily disturb an entire hospital ward. Benzodiazepines which were widely used to treat anxiety are not usually effective in the seriously disturbed patient unless given in very large doses and this inevitably results in extreme drowsiness. The aim of treatment in the examples listed above is to reduce agitation without producing excessive sedation.

Phenothiazines

This is a most important group of drugs and includes chlorpromazine, promazine, trifluoperazine and fluphenazine. One other member of the group, prochlorperazine, has litle sedative action and is used as an antiemetic.

Chlorpromazine

This drug, in addition to being a very efficient tranquillising agent, has a large number of different actions. The most important of these is that chlorpromazine has strong antiemetic properties. It is therefore given as symptomatic treatment to patients who are vomiting or feeling nauseated. It is sometimes given with a drug which is known to cause vomiting in a particular patient in the hope that this unpleasant side effect will be averted. The main use of the drug, however, is in the management of psychotic patients whose mental illnesses are characterised by marked agitation and anxiety. Chlorpromazine and its derivatives have proved invaluable in this field and have revolutionised the treatment of schizophrenic patients. In large doses the drug allows them to attain a state of remission whereby they can live outside of a mental hospital (to which they would otherwise be committed for life) and to continue in useful employment.

Chlorpromazine is a valuable adjunct in potentiating the analgesic effect of morphine and its derivatives. A usual initial dose is 25 mg thrice daily but psychiatric patients often require doses of the order of 1 g daily.

Chlorpromazine can cause a skin rash in susceptible individuals who come into contact with the drug. If you have previously had a contact dermatitis it is wise to use gloves when handling chlorpromazine tablets or when preparing a solution of this drug for intramuscular injection.

Side effects of chlorpromazine

Chlorpromazine has five main side effects which you should know. They are:

1. Liability to cause postural hypotension
2. Drug-induced jaundice
3. Drug-induced Parkinson's disease
4. Interference with temperature regulation.

Chlorpromazine should not be given to patients in whom the systolic blood pressure is less than 100 mm of mercury because of its tendency to cause hypotension.

The drug induces the development of jaundice in about 1 patient in every 100 given chlorpromazine. The condition is not usually serious for it clears up when chlorpromazine is stopped. The cause of the jaundice is not related to liver parenchymal cell damage but rather to a toxic effect of the drug on the bile canaliculi.

Parkinson's disease is another side effect in patients receiving treatment with chlorpromazine. Rigidity and tremor tend to clear up readily when the drug is stopped.

Because of the effect of chlorpromazine on temperature regulation, hypothermia may be induced particularly in the elderly in cold weather.

The drug often causes marked drowsiness.

Promazine

This drug is essentially similar in its actions to chlorpromazine. It is more prone to cause hypotension but less toxic to the liver.

Trifluoroperazine and fluphenazine

These agents share similar properties. They have less of a depressant action than chlorpromazine. All of these drugs are less likely to cause hepatic damage than chlorpromazine but they all have a propensity to induce facial tics, muscular twitchings and Parkinson's disease. On occasion this effect can be very severe and the patient's muscles go into spasm necessitating withdrawal of the drug.

All of these agents have antiemetic properties.

Fluphenazine is available in two long-acting forms which are especially useful for the long term control of schizophrenic patients: fluphenazine decanoate and fluphenazine ethanoate. These drugs act for approximately 4 and 2 weeks respectively following intramuscular injection.

Miscellaneous

Haloperidol and trifluperidol

These are potent tranquillisers which are sometimes used in the treatment of schizophrenia and mania. The dose is very variable and patients on very high doses are prone to develop a Parkinson-like state which can be severe.

DRUGS USED IN THE TREATMENT OF DEPRESSION

Everyone has experienced depression at one time or another. Loss of a close relative, failure in an important examination or happenings of this sort induce a feeling of depression which may last for a long time. In fact, to fail to be depressed at such times would be abnormal. There are individuals, however, who become deeply depressed for no obvious reason or who remain depressed for years after an incident which would cause a normal person to be depressed for weeks or a few months at the most. When psychiatrists use the term 'depression' it is this abnormal state of lowness of spirits to which they are referring. Many psychiatrically depressed patients may feel so miserable that they wish to end it all by taking their own lives and some of them do just that. Much attention has been directed in recent years towards identifying a biochemical basis for depression. No definite conclusions have been reached but there is some evidence that the concentration in the brain of a number of chemicals known as amines may be important. The two effective groups of antidepressants in use, the tricyclic group and related compounds and the monoamine oxidase inhibitors elevate the levels of brain amines and it is possible that this is the basis of their efficacy.

Tricyclic antidepressants

As with the beta-blocking drugs, development in recent years has resulted in the production of a vast number of new tricyclic drugs (so named because their chemical structure contains three rings). There is no convincing evidence that the newer tricyclic drugs are superior to the older ones so our discussion is confined to the more established compounds that you will see in common use.

Amitriptyline, nortriptyline and imipramine

These are the three drugs which have been in use for the longest time. As they are rather similar in structure and effect, they will be considered together. They are fairly potent agents in the treatment of depression and it is likely that early treatment in general practice with these agents prevents a number of cases of severe depression which would otherwise have required more intensive therapy in hospital. As stated earlier, the exact mode of action of these drugs is not known but they may act by increasing the levels of amines in the brain by blocking re uptake by the cerebral cells.

Protriptyline

Protriptyline is a relatively stimulant antidepressant and so it is less suited to the treatment of patients who are agitated as well as depressed. It is thought to be of value in elderly patients who are depressed and lethargic following a stroke.

It appears to have a quicker onset of action than imipramine and amitriptyline.

Doxepin

Doxepin is chemically related to amitriptyline. In addition to being an antidepressant, doxepin has tranquillising properties and resembles diazepam and chlordiazepoxide. It is a good treatment for the depressed anxious patient.

Side effects of the tricyclic antidepressants

All of these drugs are liable to cause adverse effects when used in therapeutic doses. Drowsiness is common shortly after commencing treatment and this usually wears off in time. It is more of a problem with amitriptyline and doxepin than with nortriptyline and protriptyline. Anticholinergic effects similar to that produced by atropine are common, resulting in complaints of dry mouth, constipation and blurred vision due to interference with the power of accommodation of the eye. Difficulty with micturition may be troublesome and urinary retention may result, particularly in elderly men with prostatic enlargement. Acute glaucoma has followed treatment with these drugs and jaundice is a rare side effect. Particularly worrying is the suggestion that these agents, and in particular amitriptyline, may produce cardiac arrhythmias and sudden death. If this in fact happens it is almost certainly a very rare event. Although this is a formidable list of side effects, these drugs are safe when used properly and they are very useful tools in the management of a most distressing condition.

Monoamine oxidase inhibitors

These drugs act by blocking the enzymes responsible for the breakdown of certain cerebral amines. They were commonly used before the advent of the tricyclic antidepressants but their use has declined sharply because of serious side effects. These drugs interact with a remarkable number of other drugs and also certain food and drinks, such as cheese, Bovril and red wine. The high content of an amino acid called tyramine in these foods results in rapid accumulation of amines within the nervous system. This in turn leads to a rapid rise in blood pressure which may prove fatal. Monoamine oxidase inhibitors are still employed by a few psychiatrists and so long as they are experienced in their use and observe the necessary restrictions they still have a place in the management of mental illness.

Lithium

This agent is used occasionally to prevent further episodes of depression or mania (sustained elevation of mood without apparent cause) in patients with depression.

This is a case in which regular measurement of the concentration of drug in the blood is important. The dosage of lithium is adjusted in each individual case to provide a fairly precise concentration within the blood. This ensures a therapeutic response that avoids toxicity. Side effects of lithium vary from mild nausea and tremor to confusion, and coma if the concentration in the blood is very high. Lithium impairs the power of the kidney to concentrate urine, so polyuria and polydipsia are common. Rarely underactivity of the thyroid gland and goitre may develop.

DRUGS USED IN THE TREATMENT OF EPILEPSY

Epilepsy may be defined as spontaneous recurring seizures caused by sudden and excessive discharge of electrical activity in the grey matter of the brain. This may result from an easily identified cause such as a depressed fracture, birth injury or a scar left by meningitis. In many cases routine investigations fail to reveal a specific cause, but treatment is very important. In the past, people suffering from epilepsy were frequently regarded as dull-witted, helpless individuals. In some cases epilepsy is in fact accompanied by mental deficiency but the majority of patients with seizures are of average intelligence and should be able to lead completely normal and useful lives if their seizures are properly controlled. It is very sad that in the past lack of understanding frequently led to either ineffective treatment or unnecessary combinations of toxic drugs which severely impaired the patient's intelligence, reinforcing the belief that epileptics are dull-witted. Modern therapy emphasises the importance of using as few drugs as possible in the most effective manner.

In simple terms, there are four types of seizures.

(1) **Grand mal (tonic clonic) seizures.** These are the classical seizures in which the patient lets out a cry, becomes rigid and then exhibits uncontrolled contractions of the major muscle groups. The patient is often apnoeic and cyanosed during the tonic (rigid) phase and tongue biting and incontinence are common. The drug of choice in this condition is phenytoin. Alternative drugs are carbamazapine and sodium valproate which are popular in children because of the toxicity of phenytoin. Phenobarbitone and primidone are also effective but are less often used nowadays because of their tendency to produce drowsiness.

(2) **Temporal lobe (psychomotor) seizures.** The temporal lobe of the brain is concerned with perception and memory. During the seizures originating from this area the patient may experience disturbances of memory, taste and smell and sometimes vivid hallucinations. The individual is uncommunicative and may exhibit unusual and at times violent behaviour. For this reason the condition is sometimes mistaken for psychiatric illness. Whereas grand mal seizures seldom occur with a frequency greater than four or five per week, temporal lobe attacks can occur up to 20 or more times in a day. The frequency of this condition is underestimated and patients with classical epilepsy often experience frequent temporal lobe attacks as well. These seizures respond to phenytoin but the drug of choice is carbamazapine.

(3) **Petit mal epilepsy (absences).** Petit mal consists of brief and often frequent attacks in which the patient suddenly stops whatever activity he or she has been indulging in and becomes completely blank. There is complete lack of communication with the surroundings. Following recovery (the attacks are very short) the patient is unaware that anything untoward has happened. This kind of epilepsy occurs in young children and it is usual for them to grow out of it. They may go on to develop other types of seizure later. True petit mal seizures are rare in adults but temporal lobe attacks may appear similar and are often mistaken for them. The distinction is important as treatment is different. The drugs of choice in petit mal epilepsy are ethosuximide and sodium valproate.

(4) **Focal (partial) seizures.** In this type of seizure only part of

the body is affected and the patient may for instance exhibit uncontrolled twitching of an arm or a leg. It is possible to talk to the patient during the attack but the seizure may progress to a full blown grand mal fit at which point other parts of the body will be affected and communication is impossible. The drugs of choice in focal attacks are sodium valproate and clonazepam.

Phenytoin

This is the most effective drug in grand mal seizures. Its precise mode of action is not known. It is usually given in a dose of between 200 and 400 mg per day and as it is slowly absorbed into and slowly excreted from the body it may be given as a single dose before bed. The best results are achieved with phenytoin when the concentration of the drug in the blood is kept within fairly precise limits. When the concentration is below this therapeutic range control of seizures may be poor and when it rises too high side effects are extremely common. Individual patients require individual amounts of drug to achieve this aim and it is not uncommon to find that some require unusual doses, for instance 225 mg or 375 mg per day for the best results. Side effects are fairly common and may be serious. Ataxia (unsteadiness of gait) and tremor will occur if the concentration of the drug in the blood is high. Double vision may occur. In severe cases of phenytoin poisoning the patient may become comatose. Skin rashes sometimes develop and may be severe. An unusual side effect is hyperplasia (overgrowth) of the gums and lips and in long standing toxicity in children the entire appearance of the face may be altered. Megaloblastic anaemia due to folic acid deficiency rarely occurs, and the drug induces hirsutism (excess facial and body hair) in some patients.

Sodium valproate

This drug is fairly new but has been increasingly used in epilepsy. It is particularly popular in children and is very effective in the treatment of petit mal. In adults it may be successful on its own in grand mal seizures, or it may be used in combination with another drug, for instance phenytoin, if that drug alone has not completely controlled the seizures. The dosage is very variable and ranges from 400 to 2000 mg or more per day. Side effects are fairly uncommon, the main ones being nausea, tremor and transient loss of hair.

Carbamazepine

This drug is also used in the painful conditon trigeminal neuralgia. It is effective treatment for grand mal seizures and is particularly useful for the control of temporal lobe attacks. Like sodium valproate it is often used in children because it is less toxic than phenytoin. Dosage varies from 400 to 1600 mg per day. Side effects may occur at high dosage and consist mainly of drowsiness and ataxia.

Phenobarbitone

This is the time honoured remedy in grand mal epilepsy. It is becoming used less often as it is more likely to produce drowsiness than some of the newer anticonvulsants. It is probably not quite as effective as phenytoin in the treatment of grand mal epilepsy. As a general rule new patients should probably receive one of the other drugs, but of course older patients who have been well controlled for years by phenobarbitone should continue to receive it. The main side effects are drowsiness and depression and this may not be apparent until the patients notice how well they fell when the drug is stopped. As with the other barbiturates skin rashes may occur and megaloblastic anaemia due to folic acid deficiency is a rare complication.

Primidone

This drug is closely related to the barbiturates and in fact the body converts it to phenobarbitone. For this reason the two drugs should not be given together. It is probably no more effective than phenobarbitone used alone and is not a 'first choice' drug in new patients. Side effects are similar to the barbiturates.

Ethosuximide

Ethosuximide is a member of a chemically related class of drugs known as succinimides. It is relatively free of serious side effects and is therefore the drug of choice for controlling petit mal in you children. The drug is usually given in a small dose working up to a maintenance dose which varies from 1 to 1.5 g per day in divided doses depending on the individual response of the child. Occasionally ethosuximide may cause gastric irritation with vomiting. Drowsiness may develop in children taking the drug.

DRUGS USED IN THE TREATMENT OF PARKINSON'S DISEASE

Parkinson's disease is a complex condition with a number of different causes. This disease is manifested by a characteristic tremor of the hands and other parts of the body. Rigidity of muscles also develops and can be recognised by the experienced eye at a glance because facial rigidity gives these patients an appearance of impassivity which makes them superficially appear rather alike. Patients with Parkinson's disease don't smile when you make a joke: it is not that they do not appreciate humour but rather that the ability to make normal facial expressions spontaneously is denied them. You will be able to discover for yourself how much we all depend on receiving signals from each other's faces during conversation when you speak to your patients with severe Parkinsonism. Initially you will feel that it is difficult to establish rapport with them and this difficulty is precisely because the patient does not smile readily or indicate what he is feeling with his facial expression. This is not to say that he does not have feelings, the reverse is indeed the case, some patients being very emotional. For patients with this disease therefore a special effort in communicating is needed.

In advanced disease there is rigidity in walking and this combined with tremor produces a peculiar rapid shuffle when walking. Increased salivation also occurs.

The features of the disease result from abnormalities in the basal ganglia, the part of the brain which controls the regulation of movement. In the basal ganglia there are two systems which balance each other. In one the chemical transmitter of nerve messages is acetylcholine, in the other it is the substance dopamine.

In Parkinson's disease the latter system is defective because dopamine levels are low and the acetylcholine system is correspondingly overactive. Drugs used to treat the disease thus work in one of two ways: they either reduce the activity of the acetylcholine system (anticholinergic drugs) or they enhance the dopamine system (dopamine enhancing drugs).

The aim of treatment is to reduce rigidity and so increase mobility. In general, tremor responds less well to therapy.

Dopamine enhancing drugs

The main drug in this class is levodopa. Amantadine may also work by enhancing dopamine levels in the basal ganglia and other drugs are currently being developed.

Levodopa

This is a precursor of dopamine to which it is converted in the brain. It represents a major advance in the treatment of Parkinsonism.

Dosage is built up slowly from 0.5 g daily till the maximum tolerated dose is reached (around 4 g daily in divided doses). The biggest drawback to attaining a satisfactory dose is that levodopa may induce nausea and vomiting. The drug should be given after food.

Rigidity and poverty of facial expression are improved most by levodopa and to a lesser extent, tremor. Full benefit may take 4 to 8 weeks to accrue although improvement may be noted as early as one week. Patients with Parkinson's disease of less than 10 years' duration benefit most. Long-term treatment (over 3 years) may bring a relapse of symptoms.

Side effects include nausea, vomiting, involuntary movements of the head, tongue or lips and choreoathetosis (a twisting writhing motion of the limbs). These are seen at the higher dose levels. Postural hypotension also occurs. Patients may become confused, excited and sleep less well. Hallucinations may require withdrawal of the drug although some patients are able to accept hallucinations as part of the price they pay for improvement.

Anticholinergic drugs may be used in combination with levodopa.

Levodopa/Carbidopa combinations

A number of proprietary drugs contain a mixture of levodopa

and carbidopa. This latter agent prevents breakdown of levodopa in the body and therefore allows more to enter the brain.
For this reason the total dose of levodopa used is reduced as are
the side effects. Most patients who respond to levodopa now
receive such a combination.

Amantadine

Unexpectedly a patient with Parkinson's disease treated for a
viral illness with amantadine was found to display improvement
in his rigidity. Amantadine is now realised to be a valuable
adjunct in Parkinson's disease.

The dose is 100 mg once or twice daily.

Side effects are uncommon in the doses recommended.

Anticholinergic drugs

These are agents which oppose the action of acetylcholine. They
reduce tremor and to a lesser extent improve rigidity. These
drugs produce dryness of the mouth (acceptable to the patient
with Parkinson's disease since excess salivation is a feature of his
disease).

Atropine

This is taken orally and often patients develop tolerance to it so
that the dose has to be progressively increased for the drug to be
effective. Blurring of vision due to impairment of the power of
accommodation often occurs.

Benzhexol and orphenadrine

These drugs are the anticholinergic agents used most commonly
in Parkinson's disease. In a few patients tremor may also be
improved. In addition, these drugs often induce a marked
feeling of euphoria in the patient. Both benzhexol and orphena-
drine are given initially in feel small dose and the dose is
increased rapidly to the limit of the patient's tolerance.

Other drugs young you may see used occasionally in the
treatment of patients with Parkinson's disease are benztropine,
procyclidine and ethopropazine.

DRUGS USED IN THE TREATMENT OF MIGRAINE

This is one of the commonest neurological disorders. It is characterised by intermittent and often severe headache which is frequently unilateral and accompanied by visual upsets, vomiting and occasionally transient loss of power or sensation in a limb. It is thought that an attack of migraine frequently starts with constriction of one of the cerebral arteries. The resulting ischaemia liberates substances such as histamine and serotonin which are thought in turn to produce intense vasodilatation and headache. The four main lines of treatment are: simple analgesics; drugs to prevent the vasodilatation; drugs to antagonise the action of serotonin; and preventive treatment with clonidine.

Simple analgesics

Aspirin and paracetamol are equally effective in the treatment of migraine. They have no effect on the underlying mechanism and only provide symptomatic relief from headache. Proprietary preparations often use combinations of these drugs, sometimes with the addition of caffeine. There is no evidence that these combinations are more effective than either drug used alone and they are certainly more expensive. Analgesics are discussed in more detail in Chapters 7 and 8.

Vasoconstrictor drugs

Ergotamine tartrate is often effective in the acute attack and presumably acts by diminishing the intense vasodilatation which produces headache. It may be given subcutaneously for rapid effect in a severe attack but is often administered orally at the first warning of a migrainous episode. Ergotamine may produce vasoconstriction of arteries in other parts of the body, particularly if used in excessive doses. Peripheral ischaemia and gangrene may result, particularly if the patient already has arterial disease. It should be avoided in these patients and must never be given in pregnancy as its stimulates uterine contraction.

Histamine and serotonin antagonists

Methysergide, a drug which antagonises the actions of histamine and serotonin, was found to be successful in preventing attacks, but it fell into disuse when an unusual and serious side effect known as retroperitoneal fibrosis developed in some patients. More recently a drug known as pizotifen, which antagonises the action of serotonin, has been found to be effective in some patients. It appears to be safe but its place in the management of migraine is not yet established.

Preventive therapy

In some patients it is possible to identify certain foodstuffs which precipitate attacks and in these cases the most effective therapy is avoidance. Where there is no obvious precipitating cause, therapy with clonidine used in lower doses than in the treatment of hypertension (see Ch. 3) may occasionally be effective. Its mode of action in this situation is not known.

7

Drugs used in the treatment of pain

PAIN

A patient recovering from an accident or surgery or dying of cancer has a right to expect adequate pain relief from doctors and nurses. Unfortunately this is not achieved in every case. Often this is due to very genuine variation in the way that different people will respond to pain. At other times it is due to failure to provide the right quantity and combination of drugs. At present a great deal of research is going on into the exact mechanisms by which pain is produced and appreciated at the cerebral cortex. Hopefully a better understanding of these mechanisms will allow us to produce new drugs and use them to greater advantage. The following section discusses the broad management of different situations in which pain arises. The individual drugs which are utilised in pain relief will be discussed later.

Management of specific problems

Acute pain

This may range from mild pain of a tension headache to the severe pain experienced following an accident or surgery. Relief

153

must be rapid and adequate but not produce unwanted side effects such as vomiting or risk of addiction.

Headache. Headache is probably the most commonly experienced pain and results in the consumption of vast quantities of analgesics every year. Tension of the posterior cervical muscles is a very common cause and self medication with aspirin or paracetamol is probably a perfectly satisfactory arrangement. Understanding of the cause of headache is clearly important as in some cases there may be a true element of depression which may respond to antidepressant therapy. Rarely headache indicates truly organic disease although you may be surprised to hear that it does not result from high blood pressure nearly as often as most people think. Serious causes of headache, in particular intracranial tumours, are uncommon but must be suspected if headache is persistent, and is associated with other complaints. It is important that the patient with recurring tension headache is not treated at an early stage with potent narcotic derivatives as this carries with it a high risk of addiction in the long run. The treatment of migraine is considered in detail in Chapter 6.

Postoperative pain. The degree of pain complained of following the same operation varies widely from one individual to another, probably because of differences in personality and also true differences in the appreciation of pain. This sort of variation cannot be measured objectively. Because of this it is worth remembering that pain is what the patient feels and that only the patient can estimate either the severity of the pain or the relief provided by drugs. Postoperative pain is very severe and morphine, diamorphine and pethidine are by far the most commonly used drugs for its relief. No other group of agents seems to provide the same combination of analgesia and improved wellbeing. Fear of causing addiction often leads to these drugs being given too infrequently and in inadequate dosage. It is very rare for addiction to occur over the short period over which postoperative pain relief is most necessary. As it is particularly important to avoid vomiting postoperatively, an antiemetic such as prochlorperazine is often prescribed in addition to an analgesic.

Myocardial infarction. The pain of a heart attack is often severe and associated with great anxiety and a sense of impending death. Because of this either morphine or diamorphine is usually given. As an addition to providing pain relief they reduce the sense of fear. As in the postoperative situation, the use of an antiemetic drug may be necessary.

Labour. The management of pain in labour is a specialised area which it would be inappropriate to go into in detail. Drugs used include a mixture of the anaesthetic gas nitrous oxide and air (entonox) and pethidine. It must be remembered that any drug given to the mother will tend cross the placenta and may cause respiratory depression of the fetus. Epidural anaesthesia is becoming more common. Psychological factors, such as relief of anxiety, are probably as important as the drugs prescribed.

Chronic pain. This may be severe and debilitating. When it is due to disease which is likely to be rapidly fatal the risk of addiction is unimportant and narcotic drugs can be freely pre-scribed. When chronic or recurring pain is due to a benign condition then its management becomes very difficult and addiction to these agents becomes common.

Terminal care. Pain experienced by patients dying of cancer is often aggravated by their fear and by depression as well as by such physical problems as nausea, vomiting, constipation or difficulty in swallowing. Those who become skilled in the care of the dying are able to create an atmosphere which assuages the distress of patients and their relatives and this may be as import-ant as the medication in relieving symptoms. Whether the analgesic required is a mild one or an opiate, the same principle applies, that it should be given regularly. It is useless to wait until the patient complains of pain and then give an analgesic as this merely allows the pain to build up and makes the management more difficult as well as undermining the patient's faith in the ability of the staff to help him or her. The drug chosen should be given at least 4-hourly, and maybe more frequently, in such doses that the patient is never in discomfort. Previous pain is forgotten and there is no escalation of distress. Many patients with malignant disease can be managed for a surprising length of time with a simple analgesic such as aspirin or paracetamol. When simple remedies fail, a more powerful analgesic such as oral pethidine or the widely used Brompton's cocktail (see below) may be required. When the dose of morphine or diamor-phine reaches high levels it may be necessary to administer the drug by injection. The phenothiazine tranquillisers, for instance chlorpromazine, appear to potentiate the action of morphine and similar analgesics and they are often added to the treatment

Other drugs which may supplement the action of analgesics include diazepam and corticosteroids. For the pain of bone or nerve infiltration radiotherapy or nerve block are required. In extreme cases cordotomy (ablation of the pain tracts in the spinal cord) may be considered.

ANALGESICS IN COMMON USE

An analgesic is a drug which diminishes pain. It is important that you appreciate the difference between this and an antiinflammatory drug which actually reduces the inflammatory process which may be the cause of pain. Antiinflammatory drugs are discussed fully in Chapter 8. Analgesic drugs seem to act by diminishing appreciation of pain within the central nervous system. They are divided into two groups, the first group is the simple analgesics which we use for the treatment of mild to moderate pain. The second group are the narcotic drugs which are used for the treatment of severe pain.

SIMPLE ANALGESICS

Aspirin

Aspirin is still the most widely used analgesic for the treatment of minor aches and pains and is of course widely available without prescription. In fact its mode of action is not clearly defined. It acts centrally by diminishing appreciation of pain but also owes some of its analgesic action to a peripheral effect at the site of pain production. It is particularly useful for the treatment of musculoskeletal pain, headache, toothache and dysmenorrhoea but seems less effective for the treatment of pain originating in the gastrointestinal or urinary tract. In higher doses it has a true anti-inflammatory effect. The most common adverse effect is gastric irritation, which does not occur as often as many people believe. Aspirin is discussed in greater detail in Chapter 8. Self-poisoning with aspirin may result in a severe metabolic disturbance.

Paracetamol

This is a simple analgesic which acts centrally and seems to have no true anti-inflammatory action. It has the advantage over aspirin that it is less inclined to cause gastric upset. The usual dose is 500 to 750 mg 4 to 6-hourly. There seems to be no advantage in increasing the dose beyond this. Self-poisoning may result in severe liver damage.

Mixed preparations

A number of proprietary drugs contain combinations of aspirin and paracetamol with other compounds such as codeine, dihydrocodeine and dextroproproxyphene. These last three drugs are morphine derivatives with much reduced potency, but when used in combination they genuinely increase the efficacy of simple analgesics. Combinations of aspirin and paracetamol with each other or with other agents such as caffeine have no advantages over aspirin or paracetamol used alone and are frequently more expensive. The most commonly used combination preparation is probably Distalgesic which contains paracetamol and dextroproproxyphene. This is relatively safe but if taken in overdosage carries the dual risk of paracetamol-induced liver damage and narcotic overdose (see below). It is a good rule to always identify the exact nature and dose of the constituents of any combination preparation which you give to a patient.

NARCOTIC ANALGESICS

A few definitions may be of some value before discussing narcotics and related substances. A *narcotic* may be defined as a drug which induces in the patient, drowsiness, sleep, stupor or insensibility and may produce drug dependence. It is obvious that drowsiness, sleep, stupor and insensibility are all manifestations in greater or lesser degree of the same thing, namely loss of consciousness.

An *analgesic* is a drug which results in the abolition of the sensation of pain. This is slightly different from an anaesthetic. An *anaesthetic* is a substance which results in the abolition of all modalities of sensation. For example, morphine which is an analgesic drug makes the patient unable to appreciate the sensation of pain although he can still appreciate the sensation of touch or of heat. Lignocaine however, is a local anaesthetic. This means that if lignocaine is injected locally into the skin or into a nerve, the patient will be able to appreciate neither the sensation of pain nor touch nor heat in that part of the skin or in that nerve.

The narcotic drugs may be divided up quite conveniently into two groups of substances. The first group consists of drugs which have sedative or hypnotic actions. The barbiturates are examples of narcotic drugs with sedative and hypnotic properties. These drugs are discussed in Chapter 6.

The second group of narcotics is made up of drugs with analgesic effects such as morphine and pethidine. As you will be aware simple analgesic drugs (such as aspirin) are not habit forming and are therefore not classified as narcotics. Most potent analgesic drugs, however, are narcotics.

Opium

This drug occurs naturally and has been known to the Chinese for many thousands of years. It is prepared from a special poppy (*Papaver somniferum*—which is the Latin for 'the sleep-bringing poppy'). The juice squeezed from the unripe seed capsule of this poppy is rich in opium. The main active ingredient of opium is morphine and there is a larger number of other substances in opium besides morphine which have a much weaker action, such as codeine. The drug is still used today as 'chalk and opium mixture' to relieve diarrhoea (see actions of morphine).

Morphine

Morphine is the principal active ingredient of opium. It is one of the most valuable drugs which we possess and it has a variety of actions apart from its capacity to relieve severe pain. It is important that you be familiar with the actions and uses of morphine. The drug can be given by oral administration but often the patient who requires morphine is too ill for this route to be used. In addition, the drug is not satisfactorily absorbed following oral administration. For these reasons parenteral administration is usually employed.

Actions of morphine

If you know the actions of morphine its therapeutic uses and side effects immediately become obvious. The actions of morphine are:

1. It acts as a sedative
2. It acts as an analgesic
3. It depresses the cough reflex
4. It stimulates the vomiting centre
5. It depresses the respiratory centre
6. It causes contraction of the smooth muscle sphincters of the alimentary tract
7. It causes sweating
8. It causes constriction of the pupils
9. Morphine is a drug of addiction.

Sedative action of morphine

Patients who are in extreme agony due to a disease such as myocardial infarction or an injury such as loss of a limb are understandably anxious. Their anxiety is obvious at a glance. They are apprehensive and restless. Morphine is a splendid drug to give these patients for in addition to relieving pain it alleviates fear and allays anxiety. It thus gives what no amount of explanation can give at this stage of illness: peace of mind. One of the great advantages of morphine is that it does not, in normal circumstances and in normal dosage, act as a hypnotic. This means that your patient remains conscious after you have given him the drug. Some patients, however, may have been suffering pain for a long time before treatment with morphine becomes available. These patients may not have slept for many hours because of pain and distress. You will often notice that shortly after a morphine injection patients of this kind drop quietly off into a sound and untroubled sleep as their pain is relieved and their fears allayed.

Analgesic action of morphine

It is not known exactly how morphine acts to produce such a profound relief of pain. The drug seems to exert its effect on pain sensitive regions in the brain. It does not abolish pain but rather makes the patient's perception of it different. The dose of morphine required to produce analgesia varies very much from patient to patient. Although the dose range is stated by many to be 8 to 20 mg, the truth of the matter is that the correct dose of morphine is that which is effective in relieving the patient's appreciation of pain. Some patients require much more than the theoretical maximum dose of morphine before their pain is relieved, while others require surprisingly little of the drug for analgesic effect.

Stimulation of the vomiting centre

There is in the brain a higher centre which controls the act of vomiting. If the activity of this centre is stimulated, patients will vomit and if it is depressed, vomiting is less likely to occur. Some drugs stimulate this centre in a few patients. Morphine stimulates it in about one-third of all patients given the drug and causes them to vomit. In a further third of patients given morphine some degree of nausea is experienced. From this you can see that morphine very commonly induces either nausea or vomiting. Apart from the distress it causes to patients, this effect of morphine is undesirable in many situations in clinical practice. For example, it is undesirable to have a patient who has recently sustained a myocardial infarction leaning out of bed with his whole body shaking with the strain of retching. For this reason morphine is sometimes given to patients with another drug such as promazine which depresses the activity of the vomiting centre in the hope that vomiting or nausea may be avoided.

Respiratory centre depression

Morphine directly suppresses the activity of the respiratory centre in the brain. This means that patients given the drug breathe more slowly and that individual breaths are shallow. Usually this is of little consequence. In patients with chronic respiratory disease, whose breathing is laboured and inefficient and who have little respiratory reserve, this action of morphine may have the gravest results. Patients with severe chronic bronchitis and emphysema have been tipped into the state of irreversible respiratory failure leading to coma and death following a single injection of morphine.

Occasionally doctors have great difficulty in distinguishing cardiac asthma (left ventricular failure) from bronchial asthma.

Yet it is very important to make the correct diagnosis between these two conditions. Morphine, as is discussed later in this chapter, is the drug of choice for the treatment of cardiac asthma while it is absolutely contra-indicated in patients with bronchial asthma. Here the depression of the respiratory centre which morphine induces may prove fatal to a patient who needs every breath he can muster.

Morphine and contraction of smooth muscle sphincters

Morphine causes smooth muscle sphincters to contract. In older people this may lead to retention of urine because of contraction of the muscle sphincters of the bladder. Acute retention of urine is especially liable to occur in elderly men given this drug because many men have enlargement of the prostate gland which itself causes difficulty with micturition. Often the effect of morphine added to the effect of prostatic gland hypertrophy is sufficient to cause an acute urinary retention. You should always be on the look-out for this complication of morphine treatment. Any elderly man who complains of abdominal discomfort or fullness should be suspect. It is always a wise move to note how much urine is passed by your elderly patients who are receiving morphine. Sometimes a full bladder may cause bizarre behaviour in the very elderly especially if they are somewhat disorientated (as many old people are in hospital). Any aged person who becomes restless or querulous after a morphine injection may be in the process of developing acute urinary retention. This is a point worth remembering.

If morphine is given to a patient suffering from biliary colic it may initially relieve his pain but later intensify it or at least render his chances of passing the stone much less. The reason for this is that the drug may induce spasm of the sphincter of Oddi where the bile duct passes into the duodenum. A further rise in intrabiliary pressure may result and this may cause the patient still further pain. This is therefore a theoretical reason for not using morphine in these patients. In practice however most patients with biliary colic obtain relief when morphine is given, and it is usually given with an antispasmodic such as atropine.

The effect of morphine on smooth muscle sphincters in the bowel is to induce constipation. The drug is therefore valuable in the symptomatic treatment of diarrhoea.

Other actions of morphine

The sweating which morphine induces is not of clinical importance. It is a lay person's common misconception that it is possible to tell a morphine addict because the pupils are constricted (or dilated). This is not so. It is true that morphine causes constriction of the pupils but this effect is transient. In addition, many other factors cause constriction of the pupils. For example, if you know someone whose pupils are chronically constricted it is quite likely that he is receiving pilocarpine drops into his eyes as a treatment for glaucoma.

Dose of morphine

A dose of 10 mg is usually adequate. The drug may be given subcutaneously, intramuscularly or intravenously. You must remember that if your patient is in a shocked or hypotensive state he may not absorb a subcutaneous or even an intramuscular injection rapidly. In some cases therefore the doctor will decide to give the drug by slow intravenous injection.

Drug dependence or drug addiction

Although the term drug dependence is preferable in some respects, the term addiction is still used.

All of the narcotics are drugs of addiction and are classified from the legal point of view as dangerous drugs.

We often use the term 'addict' in our everyday speech to mean someone who is very fond of something. We may say of friends with sweet teeth that they are chocolate addicts. When the term is used to describe someone who is addicted to or dependent on drugs, however, it has a very different meaning. A patient who is addicted exhibits three features:

1. He develops tolerance to the drug to which he is dependent
2. He develops habituation to his drug
3. He shows withdrawal symptoms if his drug is stopped.

Tolerance means that the patient is able to take large doses of the drug without upset. For example, if 100 mg of morphine were administered intravenously to a normal person, this overdose might kill him. Some morphine addicts are able to inject themselves with doses of 100 mg or more without danger. They have developed tolerance to the drug.

Habituation is the feature which comes closest to the lay person's conception of addiction. The term means that the addict is mentally dependent on the drug. He feels upset and irritable without it. Cigarette smokers (who are in reality addicted to the drug nicotine) afford a good everyday example of habituation. If you have a friend who smokes, you will often notice that in times of stress (for example immediately after a written examination) her first action is to reach for a cigarette. Anyone who has ever had a member of their family try to give up smoking will realise what the term 'habituation' means.

Withdrawal symptoms show that the addict depends on his drug not only mentally but also physically. When his drug is withheld from the morphine addict he develops physical symptoms such as shivering turns, tremors, dryness of the mouth or a desire for something sweet to eat. Withdrawal symptoms are not similar for all drugs of addiction but tend to differ from one drug to the next.

By far the greatest number of narcotic addicts in this country are doctors and nurses. These unfortunate people have perhaps yielded to an impulse when they were tired or emotionally upset in the course of their duties and helped themselves to a tablet or an injection. You must *never* take medicine of any sort from the ward stores of drugs. Two or three injections or tablets of morphine might be sufficient to start a person who has no need of morphine (from pain or illness) on the path to drug addiction. Make up your mind now that you will never take any kind of medicine unless on a doctor's prescription.

Uses of morphine and derivatives

1. The relief of pain
2. The treatment of patients in left ventricular failure
3. Cough suppression (p. 83–94)
4. The symptomatic treatment of diarrhoea (p. 25)
5. Preoperative medication.

Morphine in the relief of pain has been discussed already in this chapter.

Morphine is a most valuable drug in the treatment of left

ventricular failure. Its mode of action in this condition is by no means fully understood but it may work by helping the patient breathe more easily. Left ventricular failure can be one of the gravest of medical emergencies. Patients with this condition believe (and sometimes rightly) that they are on the point of death. The respirations are quick and shallow, the patient is grey-faced and sits propped up on pillows fighting for breath. Often, white frothy sputum occludes the trachea or main bronchi and occasionally this sputum is tinged with pink. The problem, as you are aware, in left ventricular failure is that the lungs are rigid and inelastic because the pulmonary vessels are distended with the back-log of blood which the left ventricle has failed to pump away. The rising pressure of blood in the pulmonary capillaries causes fluid to exude into the alveoli whence it is coughed up as a frothy white spit.

In this situation two effects of morphine are probably beneficial. Firstly, it calms the patient. It is common experience that if we are frightened we become conscious of our breathing. This is because our breathing has become quicker and slightly inefficient. The second useful action of morphine is to depress the sensitivity of the respiratory centre to the numerous messages with which the blood-engorged lungs are bombarding it. Each time a message arrives, the respiratory centre stimulates the lungs to breathe. This means that the patient breathes too quickly and therefore too inefficiently. Morphine by its action on the respiratory centre reduces the number of impulses to which it responds and reduces the rate of respiration thus increasing the efficiency of respiration.

The usefulness of the drug in patients with haemorrhage or as a preoperative medication is based on its capacity to relieve anxiety.

Side effects of morphine

These follow from an understanding of the actions of morphine and have already been discussed. They are:

1. The induction of nausea and vomiting in many patients given the drug
2. Depression of the activity of the respiratory centre
3. Acute rention of urine
4. Drug addiction.

Nalorphine. This is a very effective antidote to morphine. Very few drugs have specific antidotes and nalorphine has proved very useful for the treatment of morphine overdose. A patient who is unconscious with barely any respiration will respond dramatically to an injection of nalorphine, becoming conscious with improved respiration in a remarkably short space of time. An unusual feature is nalorphine has some depressant action of its own. Given in morphine overdose it blocks the morphine receptors so improving the patient. If, however, it is given to somebody who is not suffering from a morphine overdose but is unconscious for some other reason, for instance a barbiturate overdose, then the added depressant effect of nalorphine may in fact make the patient worse. For this reason it must be used with care if the diagnosis is in doubt.

Naloxone. This is a newer drug and is a highly active and very specific morphine antagonist which, unlike nalorphine, has no depressant action of its own. It is therefore a safer drug and has replaced nalorphine as the drug of choice in poisoning with morphine and other related substances. It can be given safely to the unconscious patient who is merely suspected of having a morphine overdose and if the diagnosis is correct will result in rapid and dramatic improvement. Its action is fairly short-lived and for this reason repeated injections may have to be given in order to keep the patient in a satisfactory clinical state. It is always given intravenously.

Codeine

Codeine is chemically related to morphine, its chemical name being methylmorphine. It is a very much weaker analgesic than morphine but like morphine it is a drug of addiction although it is also weaker than morphine in this respect. This drug is a stronger analgesic than aspirin. It is a useful drug for the symptomatic treatment of diarrhoea and it is a useful cough suppressant given as syrup of codeine phosphate. The effects of excess codeine are similar to the effects of morphine overdosage although obviously the dose must be much larger. Certain individuals however are susceptible, for instance patients with chronic lung or liver disease. Naloxone will reverse the effects of codeine.

Dihydrocodeine (DF 118)

This is a derivative of codeine which has greater potency. It is a very popular analgesic for moderate pain and can be given orally or intramuscularly in doses of 30 to 60 mg. Like codeine it is incorporated in small doses in a wide range of proprietary mixed analgesic preparations. Its side effects are those of any morphine derivative, constipation being a problem with chronic use. True addiction occasionally occurs and overdosage may result in coma. The effects of excess dihydrocodeine can be antagonised effectively by naloxone.

Papaveretum ('Omnopon')

This consist of a mixture of morphine and the other alkaloids of opium. It is administered parenterally. The effective therapeutic dose is usually twice that of morphine. It is doubtful if papaveretum has any distinct advantages over morphine but the drug has a time-honoured place as a premedication to operation. It is used here to allay the patient's apprehensions and fears on the morning of his operation. It is very successful in doing this as your patient will tell you if you ask him about it after the operation.

Pethidine

The best known of the synethetic narcotics with analgesic properties is the drug pethidine which has a weaker analgesic effect than morphine. It may cause less depression of the respiratory centre but it is just as likely to cause nausea and vomiting as morphine. Morphine is to be preferred to pethidine where relief from agonising pain is called for. In obstetric practice, however, pethidine is used rather than morphine because of the risks associated with inducing depression of the respiratory centre in the foetus. Pethidine can be given orally but is usually given by subcutaneous injection. You will often notice marked symptoms of euphoria in your patient after an injection of pethidine, especially if the drug was given intravenously.

Methadone

This drug is a synthetic analogue of morphine. It is better

absorbed and can thus be given orally. It causes less nausea and vomiting than morphine. Drug dependence is less severe with methadone, indeed drug addicts are often transferred to it from morphine or heroin as part of their withdrawal programme. The dose is 5 mg.

Diamorphine (Heroin)

The chemical name of this agent is di-acetyl morphine and it is changed to morphine in the body. Diamorphine is the most potent of the narcotic analgesics. It is a shorter-acting drug than morphine but seems to cause less sedation and nausea which makes it a very popular choice for the pain of myocardial infarction. It is a very powerful addictive compound and must therefore be very carefully used. A typical dose of 2.5 to 5.0 mg can be given intramuscularly or by slow intravenous injection. Diamorphine can also be given orally and is included in Brompton's mixture.

Brompton's mixture

This is a mixture of either diamorphine or morphine with cocaine. It is usually mixed with an alcohol solution to provide a more pleasant taste. Brompton's mixture is usually made up specially for each patient in the hospital pharmacy and the relative amounts of diamorphine and cocaine can be varied according to the need. A commonly used combination contains 15 mg of morphine, 10 mg of cocaine, 5 ml of spirit and 3.5 ml of syrup or honey. The alcohol base can be altered according to the taste of the patient, gin and brandy being common choices. Chlorpromazine elixir may also be added to the mixture. This combination is most effective for the chronic treatment of terminal disease and often has a dramatic effect on morale. The morphine or diamorphine very effectively diminishes pain while the mixture of cocaine and alcohol improves mood.

Pentazocine

This drug has analgesic activity midway between codeine and morphine. Addiction to pentazocine does occur but is much less of a risk than with morphine. Unlike morphine, pentazocine does not have a tranquillising effect after injection although a few patients do experience euphoria after parenteral administration of the drug.

Unwanted effects include the induction of hallucinations which can be very frightening. Palpitations, increased sweating and hypotension occur occasionally.

Pentazocine can be given orally, intramuscularly or intravenously. A typical oral dose is 50 mg.

Dextropropoxyphene

This drug resembles methadone in its chemical structure. It has analgesic activity approximately equal to that of codeine. It suppresses cough although less effectively than codeine and it also has less tendency to produce dependence.

Dextropropoxyphene may be given on its own but is more commonly given in the form of 'Distalgesic', a proprietary combination which contains 325 mg of paracetamol and 32.5 mg of dextropropoxyphene.

8

Drugs used in the treatment of rheumatic diseases

'Rheumatic diseases' is a rather vague term which is used to describe a group of diverse conditions which are all character-ised to a greater or lesser degree by pain and inflammation of the joints. Included in this group are rheumatoid arthritis, systemic lupus erythematosis, a less common condition in which many structures other than the joints are damaged, and ankylosing spondylitis in which the spinal column bears the main brunt of injury. Also included are osteoarthritis, primarily a degenerative condition but one in which inflammation around the joint may contribute to pain, and gout in which acute inflammation is precipitated by deposition of uric acid crystals within the joint. In this latter condition reduction of the concentration of uric acid in the blood is more important than anti-inflammatory therapy, but in the other conditions mentioned specific curative or preventive therapy is not available and treatment aims to pro-duce maximum reduction of inflammation, pain and disability with a minimum of side effects. Thus, although we are dealing with a group of diverse and mainly unrelated conditions the treatment of each is similar. Where genuine differences occur this will be highlighted under the discussion of individual drugs. Finally, mention must be made of rheumatic fever. This previ-ously common condition is now comparatively rare. It probably represents an abnormal response by the body to infection by the haemolytic streptococcus and although the damage to joints and heart is treated by anti-inflammatory drugs, this condition is unique amongst the rheumatic diseases in that further attacks can be prevented by long-term treatment with penicillin.

ANTI-INFLAMMATORY DRUGS

As rheumatoid arthritis is the commonest and arguably the most crippling of the true inflammatory diseases most of the following discussion with be directed towards its treatment.

Any discussion of these drugs must be prefaced with the remark that at present none of them *cures* the patient with rheumatoid arthritis. At best they provide some relief of pain, at worst they can cause serious side effects. For this reason caution is required in their use. Some of the difficulties which patients with rheumatoid arthritis find hardest to bear stem not from their disease but from the side effects of the drugs used in treatment.

A distinction must be made here between an analgesic drug which merely dulls the appreciation of pain and a true anti-inflammatory drug which reduces the inflammation which causes pain. An example of a commonly used analgesic is paracetamol. Aspirin used in low doses also acts as a simple analgesic. In high doses it has both analgesic and anti-inflammatory actions. The mode of action of most anti-inflammatory drugs is not known. Interest has recently centred around their effects on prostaglandins. These naturally occurring compounds are present throughout the body and are found in high concentrations around inflamed tissues. Some of the anti-inflammatory drugs in common use may act by inhibiting the synthesis of these prostaglandins.

Aspirin

This seemingly simple substance is in reality a complex one with a large number of different actions. The drug has three main properties:

1. It is an analgesic
2. It is an antipyretic agent: it reduces fever
3. It has some anti-inflammatory activity.

The analgesic effect of aspirin may be quite marked in some patients. When relief of pain is required throughout the day two or three tablets (600 to 900 mg) may be taken four times a day. It is a good idea to advise your patients to take aspirin after meals rather than on an empty stomach. In this way the nausea and epigastric pain which some patients experience with aspirin may be diminished.

The antipyretic effect of aspirin can be seen in any patient with a fever but is perhaps best demonstrated in patients with rheumatic fever. After 24 hours of treatment with aspirin in higher doses the pyrexia which these patients exhibit almost always begins to return to normal.

Aspirin has a mild to moderate anti-inflammatory effect which is of some value in the management of patients with rheumatoid arthritis. Joints may become less swollen after the drug is given in full doses to these patients.

Aspirin's full anti-inflammatory action is not seen until a total dose of between 4 and 8 g per day is reached in an adult. This of course requires that the patient swallows a large number of tablets and side effects are quite common. When patients are receiving large doses for a long time the blood level of aspirin is often monitored. This ensures that enough drug is being given while avoiding the serious effects associated with overdose (see below). Although aspirin used properly is effective, many patients and doctors find it rather inconvenient and favour alternative therapy.

Side effects of aspirin

These may be conveniently listed as side effects related to overdosage of aspirin and side effects which occur with therapeutic doses of the drug. The four main adverse effects of aspirin are:

1. Vertigo and deafness ⎫ Related to
2. Hyperventilation ⎬ overdosage
3. Nausea vomiting and ⎫ Occurring in
   dyspepsia ⎬ therapeutic dosage
4. Haematemesis and melaena ⎭

Vertigo. Vertigo means that the patient has the sensation that objects are spinning round him or that he himself is spinning round and round. It is a most disagreeable and frightening symptom and occurs when aspirin reaches a dangerously high level in the blood following overdosage. The treatment is to stop aspirin immediately and to put the patient to bed for a day or so until vertigo settles.

Ringing in the ears (tinnitus) and deafness occur when the levels of aspirin in the blood are very high. Like vertigo they indicate a toxic effect of aspirin on the vestibulocochlear nerve.

Hyperventilation. This side effect of aspirin treatment is seen most commonly in young children in whom it is often the first sign of overdosage with the drug. Those of you who make your careers in paediatric nursing may see hyperventilation in your young patients being treated for rheumatic fever with large doses of aspirin.

Nausea, vomiting and dyspepsia. Aspirin has a local irritant effect on the gastric mucosa whereby nausea and vomiting may be produced. Some patients experience abdominal pain after taking aspirin tablets. All of these symptoms are especially liable to occur in patients who have a gastric or a duodenal ulcer. One way to reduce the frequency of occurrence of these side effects or to reduce their severity is to prescribe aspirin tablets which have a special coating on the outside. This coating is impervious to the action of hydrochloric acid in the stomach and the tablet therefore does not dissolve. Once the tablet has passed out of the stomach, the digestive juices in the jejunum dissolve the outside coating releasing aspirin which is then absorbed.

An alternative and simpler method of reducing these side effects is to advise that aspirin be taken after and not before meals.

Haematemesis and melaena. All anti-inflammatory drugs share a tendency to irritate and inflame the stomach. Occasionally this may lead to bleeding and it is likely that patients who already have a peptic ulcer are especially at risk. Although aspirin has been given a bad name because of fears that it induces bleeding, it should be remembered that enormous quantities are consumed by the public every day and most of this is bought across the counter. Despite this, very few individuals come to any real harm and serious bleeding as a result of aspirin is very rare.

An unusual side effect of aspirin is its tendency to cause acute asthmatic attack in a few people who are genuinely allergic to it. This can sometimes be very severe.

Although much has been made of its side effects aspirin is still a very useful and comparatively safe drug. A case can be made for commencing most patients on a trial of aspirin therapy before proceeding to more complex treatment for arthritis of any form.

Paracetamol

Unlike aspirin, paracetamol has no true anti-inflammatory activity and its value in the treatment of true inflammatory diseases is therefore very limited. It is a valuable and a safe analgesic as it is not liable to cause the side effects associated with aspirin when used in therapeutic dosage for a long time. A usual analgesic dose is 1 g repeated 3 to 4 times a day. For minor aches and pains paracetamol is probably the drug of choice and is to be preferred to aspirin.

If you come to work eventually outside a hospital you may have to advise patients on the choice of a suitable analgesic for minor aches and pains which are not severe enough to take them to the doctor. Paracetamol is a useful drug to have about the home. If it is to be bought in a chemist's shop in Great Britain instruct your patients to ask for paracetamol tablets B.P. (B.P. stands for British Pharmacopeia) rather than a proprietary preparation of paracetamol such as Panadol.

Panadol tablets contain only paracetamol in the same dose as the official B.P. preparation but are some three to four times as expensive. You will find that patients are grateful for this kind of advice. Paracetamol in overdose causes liver damage which may be fatal. No more than 10 tablets a day should be taken.

Proprietary compounds

A large number of proprietary compounds contain mixtures of aspirin and paracetamol, sometimes together and sometimes in combination with small doses of other agents such as codeine and caffeine. In general there is no good evidence that these mixtures are any more effective in the treatment of rheumatic conditions than aspirin used alone. A particularly popular combination in hospital practice is 'Distalgesic' which contains paracetamol and dextroproproxyphene. This latter drug and other morphine derivatives such as codeine and dihydrocodeine (DF 118) are discussed in the chapter on the treatment of pain.

Phenylbutazone

This is an analgesic drug with quite marked anti-inflammatory effects. It sometimes provides analgesic relief in rheumatoid arthritis where aspirin has failed or where the patient was unable to tolerate aspirin. Phenylbutazone is liable to cause serious, and, on occasion, fatal side effects and for this reason it should never be given to patients with rheumatoid arthritis before a careful and unhurried trial of aspirin in full doses. Phenylbutazone is also of use in the management of pain due to osteoarthritis and ankylosing spondylitis, a painful condition of the spine which afflicts principally young men.

Side effects of phenylbutazone

This drug has a number of side effects which limit its use considerably. Some of these are:

1. Gastric irritation
2. Skin rashes
3. Fluid retention
4. Agranulocytosis
5. Interactions with other drugs.

Phenylbutazone quite often causes nausea and abdominal discomfort. Inflammation of the stomach may occur and it is possible that use of the drug has led to peptic ulceration in some patients. Gastrointestinal bleeding may result. Patients who already have a duodenal ulcer often find that their ulcer symptoms are greatly aggravated by phenylbutazone.

Skin rashes which sometimes complicate therapy with phenylbutazone are a clear indication for stopping the drug. To persist with treatment is to ask the patient to run the risk of developing exfoliative dermatitis.

Fluid retention by the kidneys sometimes occurs in patients receiving this drug. The clinical effects of this are oedema of the lower limbs. Usually the patient will complain that his shoes become too tight for him at night time. Oedema tends to gravitate to the lower limbs throughout the day and swelling of the ankles and feet is a common presenting sign of oedema for any cause.

Very rarely depression of the bone marrow resulting in thrombocytopaenia (low platelet count) or agranulocytosis (low white cell count) has developed in patients receiving phenylbutazone. In a number of cases this serious side effect has been irreversible and has resulted in death. Although this is a rare side effect of a widely used drug, phenylbutazone causes this grave reaction more often than any other drug in use, other than the cytoxic group.

Phenylbutazone is carried in plasma bound to albumin for which it has a high affinity. It may displace other drugs normally carried bound to albumin such as anticoagulants with disastrous effects (Ch. 13).

Many of the side effects of phenylbutazone are dose dependant. They may be avoided if the dose of phenylbutazone is kept to a minimum. In practice it is wise to restrict the daily dose of the drug to not more than 300 mg in patients who are being treated on a long-term basis.

Indomethacin

This is a fairly potent anti-inflammatory drug which also seems to have a central analgesic effect. It seems to owe some of its effects to inhibition of prostaglandin production around inflamed tissues. It is a rather unusual drug in that although its main use is in the treatment of rheumatic diseases it has also been found to be useful in a diverse group of conditions including premature labour, patent ductus arteriosis in neonates and a rare kidney disease known as Bartter's syndrome. The feature which is common to these conditions is that inhibition of prostaglandin production leads to improvement in each case.

Indomethacin is used in arthritis in a dose of 25 or 50 mg three times daily and it is certainly effective in reducing pain and inflammation around joints. It is a safer drug than phenylbutazone but probably leads to genuine peptic ulceration in a few individuals. The characteristics of this ulceration are that it may involve stomach and duodenum simultaneously. The ulcers are deep and liable to perforate and sometimes they are of an unusual appearance which leads to the suspicion of malignant change when a barium meal X-ray is performed. Peptic ulceration usually occurs after prolonged oral administration but may even occur when the drug is administered by suppository. Ulcers like this are probably rare but minor side effects are very common with indomethacin.

A curious feature of indomethacin is the effect which it has on the central nervous system. Complaints of headache and severe giddiness are mentioned by many patients who receive this drug. Others become anxious, restive and confused. If high doses of indomethacin are given, as many as 50 per cent of patients will experience some kind of side effect referrable to the central nervous system. These side effects may be avoided if small doses of the drug (such as 25 mg thrice daily) are employed.

Ibuprofen

This drug was the forerunner of a number of new anti-inflammatory drugs which were introduced in the hope that they would be safer than phenylbutazone and indomethacin. A fairly wide range of similar drugs is available but as ibuprofen is still the most widely used discussion will be confined to it. Ibuprofen has a moderate anti-inflammatory action in arthritis although in higher doses it may prove almost as effective as indomethacin. It is certainly a fairly safe drug and apart from a tendency to produce gastric irritation it seldom causes major problems. In the past it was given orally in a dose of 200 mg three times daily but it has been found to be more effective and apparently just as safe in a dose of 400 mg three or four times daily.

Naproxen

This is a fairly new anti-inflammatory drug. It is probably as effective as indomethacin or ibuprofen. It has no clear advantages over either drug. It is less likely to induce side effects than indomethacin.

Mefenamic acid; flufenamic acid

These two drugs which are chemically similar have weak anti-inflammatory activity. They share a propensity to cause severe diarrhoea and this limits their use.

Gold salts

Gold is most commonly administered to patients with rheumatoid arthritis as an organic salt, sodium aurothiomalate. It has been shown that this compound is of some value in arresting the disease in its active progress but the long-term results obtained by treating rheumatoid arthritis patients with gold are disappointing. Gold salts are therefore used less often than they once were. They are given by weekly intramuscular injections of 50 mg to a total of not more than 1 g. Severe side effects may occur in patients who receive gold salts. Skin rashes which may proceed to exfoliative dermatitis, diarrhoea, renal damage, hepatic damage leading to jaundice, and agranulocytosis all occur.

If you have a patient undergoing gold treatment you must test the urine for albumin before giving him his weekly injection. A routine blood examination is also performed as the appearance of proteinuria or a fall in the blood count may be the first signs of serious damage to the kidneys or bone marrow.

Penicillamine

This drug has been available for a long time and was originally used to bind and remove lead from the body in cases of poisoning. It was found that penicillamine, like gold, diminishes inflammation in rheumatoid arthritis and occasionally halts progress of the disease. Use of the drug is limited by its severe side effects which include skin rashes, bone marrow depression and kidney damage.

Chloroquine

The drug, used in the treatment of malaria and amoebic hepatitis, is occasionally of benefit in the acute phase of rheumatoid arthritis. Doses of 250 to 400 mg are required and treatment for some months if improvement is to be noted.

Chloroquine suffers from the severe disadvantage of causing damage to the cornea and retina of the eye when given over long periods. Degeneration of the retina is induced by this drug and unfortunately the process starts at the macula which is the most light sensitive portion of the retina. The visual defect produced as a side effect of chloroquine treatment is thus severe. Corneal opacities also may develop in patients receiving the drug. It is questionable whether chloroquine has any place in the routine management of patients with rheumatoid arthritis. If it is used patients should be assessed annually by an ophthalmologist.

Corticosteroid drugs

Hydrocortisone is produced by the adrenal cortex and is an important hormone which helps regulate carbohydrate metabolism and salt and water balance. In physiological quantities hydrocortisone is essential to the normal functioning of the body. In large (pharmacological) doses, hydrocortisone has profound effects on protein metabolism and exerts a more powerful anti-inflammatory action than any other drug currently available. Cortisone has an almost identical structure to hydrocortisone but lacks an essential chemical group which gives the drugs its activity. If cortisone is administered to a patient it must be converted to hydrocortisone in the liver to be active. The side effects which result from corticosteroid therapy depend on the dose and duration of therapy. For this reason younger patients who may need treatment for most of their lives are not given these drugs if at all possible. After many years of treatment the side effects of corticosteroids may be more disabling than the disease process itself. It is of course important that these drugs are not withheld if the patient is suffering from a life threatening illness or if the alternative is confinement to a wheelchair. In the elderly, rheumatoid arthritis can be a surprisingly acute and sometimes short-lived illness which can quickly cripple the patient. In this situation corticosteroids will be administered more readily to prevent the disabling results of the disease. Polymyalgia rheumatica is an unusual illness which exclusively attacks the over-60s. It is characterised by severe muscular pain and stiffness and is sometimes associated with inflammation of the arteries which can lead to cerebral thrombosis or blindness. This condition is usually sensitive to corticosteroids and prompt effective treatment is mandatory as death or severe disability can be prevented by the use of these drugs. Corticosteroids are members of a class of synthetically prepared compounds which are all chemically related and have more or less the same action. These compounds are referred to collectively as corticosteroid drugs (or steroids, for short) and differences between them are largely a matter of dosage. Hydrocortisone is used either for topical application to the skin or for intravenous administration. Prednisolone, triamcinolone, dexamethasone and betamethasone are given orally although some of these compounds are also available as preparations for topical application to the skin.

Cortisone and hydrocortisone are the least potent members of the group as far as effects on the metabolism of protein and carbohydrate are concerned. These two drugs however are much more likely than the others to cause the kidneys to retain salt and water and are thus more likely to cause high blood pressure. Prednisone and prednisolone are roughly five times as potent in the effects on protein and carbohydrate metabolism as hydrocortisone. Dexamethasone and betamethasone are approximately thirty-five times as potent as hydrocortisone.

Dosage of corticosteroid drugs

Although a wide range of preparations is available it is better to know one or two drugs really well than to try and learn about all of them. Prednisolone is probably the most commonly used corticosteroid agent. For the treatment of acute life threatening conditions it is generally administered in a dose of 60 mg or more per day. Treatment is generally started in 'divided' doses, for instance 15 mg 6-hourly and these are then progressively reduced over a period of weeks, this being dictated by the severity of the condition. Once the maintenance dose, for instance 10 to 15 mg per day, has been reached, it is better to give this as a single dose in the morning as this is less likely to suppress the adrenal glands (see below). If treatment is to be continued for a long time side effects can be reduced to a minimum by keeping the maintenance dose below 15 mg per day and if possible administering the drug on alternate days only, for instance 30 mg on alternate mornings rather than 15 mg every morning

Uses of corticosteroid drugs

Corticosteroid drugs are used in a bewildering number of diseases. The position is simplified by realising that there are basically only two uses to which these drugs may be put:

1. Physiological use
2. Pharmacological use.

Physiological uses of corticosteroid drugs. Corticosteroid drugs are used physiologically to replace the needs of the body for hydrocortisone after the operation of bilateral adrenalectomy, in Addison's disease or in patients with hypopituitarism. The drug usually used is cortisone and it is given in the small physiological doses which the adrenal glands usually secrete each day (eg. 20 to 30 mg daily).

Pharmacological uses of corticosteroid drugs. Here corticosteroid drugs are used in doses very much larger than the physiological needs of the body. These larger doses are referred to as pharmacological doses. In pharmacological dosage corticosteroid drugs modify or completely suppress the inflammatory response of the body to disease. They thus dampen down the signs of activity of many disease processes, among them rheumatoid arthritis, rheumatic fever, ulcerative colitis and the rare conditions polyarteritis nodosa and systemic lupus erythematosus. This does not mean that corticosteroid drugs *cure* these diseases. Their action in some of these conditions has been likened to giving a man (the patient) going into a raging furnace (the active disease) an asbestos suit (corticosteroid therapy). The abestos suit does *not* put out the furnace, it only makes the man less aware of the heat of the fire.

Another action of corticosteroid drugs in pharmacological dosage is to modify or suppress the allergic reactions which occur in patients with some skin diseases and in some patients with bronchial asthma. The emergency use of intravenous hydrocortisone is some patients with acute attacks of bronchial asthma may be life-saving.

Corticosteroid drugs are also sometimes used in pharmacological dosage because of their effect in suppressing the abnormal production of antibodies which characterises certain diseases, notably acquired auto-immune haemolytic anaemia and some cases of thrombocytopenic purpura. They are also used as part of a multiple drug regimen in the treatment of acute luekaemia.

Corticosteroids are used to suppress rejection following renal transplants and are also of value in reducing cerebral swelling in patients who have raised intracranial pressure, for instance in association with a cerebral tumour. The drug used in this situation is usually dexamethasone.

The uses of corticosteroid drugs in patients with rheumatoid arthritis

The place of corticosteroids in the treatment of patients with rheumatoid arthritis may be summed up in one sentence: if it is at all possible, do not give corticosteroid drugs to patients with rheumatoid arthritis. The reason for this statement will become clear when the side effects of these drugs are discussed. Many patients with rheumatoid arthritis *are* given corticosteroids. What factors force doctors to use them? Some patients continue to have pain in spite of intense treatment with anti-inflammatory drugs. In addition no drugs so far discussed are as successful as corticosteroids in relieving the stiffness of which rheumatoid arthritis sufferers complain. Corticosteroids, however, are not a *cure* for rheumatoid arthritis. Benefits produced by them tend to be short lived. They bring in their wake a train of disagreeable or dangerous side effects. The vast majority of patients given these drugs will experience one or more of these side effects.

Side effects of corticosteroid drugs

It is perhaps not surprising that corticosteroid drugs which have such profound actions on the metabolism of the body, when given in physiological dosage, should produce a vast number of side effects when used in pharmacological dosage. These may be:

1. Effects on the skin and subcutaneous fat
2. Induction of diabetes mellitus
3. Induction of hypertension
4. Osteoporosis
5. Psychosis
6. Increased liability to infections
7. Development of peptic ulceration
8. Lowered resistance to stress.

Effects on skin and subcutaneous fat. The cosmetic effects of corticosteroid drugs are markedly disfiguring. Patients develop purple striae of the skin of the thighs, buttocks, abdomen and arms. A curious kind of obesity occurs in which fat is gained round the centre of the body (trunk and abdomen) while the arms and legs are spared. A typical site for the development of a pad of fat is the nape of the neck. The appearance which results from this is kindly referred to by doctors as a 'buffalo's hump'. Swelling of the face is partly accounted for by obesity and partly by retention of water. This appearance is called 'mooning' of the face because the facies loses it normal shape and becomes totally rounded like a full moon. Acneform rashes appear on the cheeks and because of the atrophic skin which patients on corticosteroids develop, purpura and spontaneous bruising ensue.

Induction of diabetes mellitus. Corticosteroids induce the development of diabetes mellitus in some individuals. The diabetes may persist even although corticosteroid therapy is stopped. Patients who have diabetes mellitus prior to starting treatment often find that steroids upset the control of the diabetes to a marked extent.

Induction of hypertension Many patients who receive corticosteroids develop a moderate degree of hypertension. This is rarely of clinical significance but the blood pressure should always be checked daily in these patients. Hypertension is not a contra-indication to the use of corticosteroid drugs.

Osteoporosis. This side effect is clinically important because it often causes spontaneous collapse of a vertebral body of fracture of a rib in patients receiving long-term corticosteroid therapy.

Increased liability to infection. Patients on long-term corticosteroid drugs are notoriously liable to severe infection. The two commonest are septicaemia (from which patients may not recover) and tuberculosis.

In normal people the inflammatory response which develops when the body is invaded by pathogenic organisms serves two functions. Firstly, it localises the infection to prevent it spreading throughout the body and secondly it causes symptoms such as pyrexia or pain in the infected part which allows early diagnosis either by the patient himself or by his doctor.

Patients on long-term corticosteroid therapy have a diminished or absent inflammatory response because steroids have a marked anti-inflammatory action. When these patients develop an infection, it tends to spread quickly (as a septicaemia) and it tends not to be diagnosed in the early stages because of the lack of reaction on the patient's part to the infection.

Psychosis. Some patients develop psychological changes while receiving corticosteroid drugs. In many this may amount to nothing more than mild euphoria. In a few patients psychological changes may progress to a full blown psychosis. This usually only happens when very high doses, for instance 80 to 100 mg of prednisolone daily, are used.

Development of peptic ulceration. Severe peptic ulceration may develop as a consequence of long-term corticosteroid therapy and patients who already have an ulcer are liable to exacerbations. The ulcers induced by corticosteroids are dangerous in that they often tend to bleed or perforate. Perforation into the peritoneal cavity may produce an atypical and extremely dangerous form of peritonitis. The patient may display none of the usual symptoms and signs of this condition because corticosteroid drugs suppress the response of the body to inflammation.

Lowered resistance to stress. Patients who are receiving or have recently received corticosteroid therapy are liable to dangerous hypotensive collapse when faced with intercurrent illness such as pneumonia or perforation or when given an anaesthetic. Even a mild injury sustained in a road accident may cause severe collapse.

Whenever the body is stressed there is an increased demand for hydrocortisone. In health, the adrenal gland meets' this demand by secreting excess hydrocortisone and in this way the response of the body to the stressful situation is maintained. After long-term corticosteroid therapy, however, the adrenal gland is unable to secrete hydrocortisone and is unable to meet the increased demands of the body for this hormone. In fact, the only way in which these increased demands can be met is to increase the dose of the corticosteroid which the patient is receiving and to keep giving him this dose for a day or so after the stress.

You will often see patients on corticosteroid drugs or who have received corticosteroid drugs in the past being given corticosteroid 'cover' before undergoing a surgical operation. If these patients were not given increased doses of corticosteroids to cover them through their operation they might die in hypotensive collapse after even quite trivial surgical procedures.

All patients on long-term corticosteroid drugs should have a card which states the dose and type of corticosteroid drug they are receiving and the date on which treatment was started. This information lets a medical attendant who is unfamiliar with details of the patient's case-history know that corticosteroid cover is necessary should an emergency befall that patient. Many hospitals now routinely issue patients on corticosteroid therapy with a card of this sort. In some hospitals it is the nurse's responsibility for filling in details of the treatment but in most centres this task falls to the doctor.

Nursing observations to be made on patients starting treatment with corticosteroid drugs

Patients who are starting treatment with corticosteroid drugs should have the urine tested daily for glucose. A number of patients will develop glycosuria on these drugs and it is important to know about this right at the start of treatment. The blood pressure should be recorded daily. Occasionally some patients may develop extremely high blood pressure readings and it may be advisable that corticosteroids be reduced on these grounds. In view of the increased tendency to obesity and the water retention which corticosteroid drugs induce, it is as well to weigh your patients weekly. Dramatic increase in weight in the early weeks of treatment may call for a reduction in steroid dosage.

It has been said that there is no member of staff who knows the patient in a hospital ward better than the nurse. Nurses are much more in contact with patients than are doctors who may at best see the patient for five to ten minutes during a morning ward round. For this reason it is often the nurse who notices that a patient is, in a vague and ill-definable way, 'less well' than he was previously. Such observations may have the greatest relevance to patients on long-term corticosteroid drugs. These patients may develop septicaemia, pneumonia, peritonitis or internal haemorrhage without necessarily exhibiting any of the clinical signs of symptoms such as pyrexia, cough, pain or pallor commonly associated with these conditions. A patient who suddenly looks iller than he was (although he may make no complaint) is worthy of comment to a senior colleague or a doctor. A simple observation on your part such as this may lead to early recognition of a potentially fatal condition.

AN OUTLINE OF THE TREATMENT OF RHEUMATOID ARTHRITIS

Rheumatoid arthritis may vary from the very mild condition requiring use of simple analgesics and mild anti-inflammatory drugs to a severe life-threatening illness which involves many tissues in the body outside the joints. The progressive crippling variety of the disease is best managed by the experienced rheumatologist who knows the limitations of the drugs, how best to use them, and most important when to enlist the help of an orthopaedic surgeon to perform synovectomy or later, reconstructive surgery. As you will have realised, the range of drugs now available is baffling, but to put in simple terms a trial of aspirin is probably worthwhile for any new case of rheumatoid arthritis. Mild cases of the condition are usually easily controlled by this or by one of the anti-inflammatory drugs such as ibuprofen, naproxon or indomethacin. More severe cases may warrant a trial of gold or penicillamine therapy. This is best managed by somebody experienced in the use of these drugs because of their frequent toxic effects. The benefits of this form of therapy are often delayed and in the interim most physicians will tend to avoid corticosteroids if possible. If the alternative is loss of livelihood and a future confined to a wheelchair then steroids are usually given. In a rheumatoid patient it is best to start with a low dose, if possible on alternate days, as this will greatly reduce the chances of serious long-term toxicity.

DRUGS USED IN THE TREATMENT OF PATIENTS WITH GOUT

Gout, a disorder characterised by high levels of uric acid in the blood, acute attacks of painful arthritis and deposition of uric acid crystals in the tissues (known as 'tophi') is a potentially curable disease. It is possible with correct treatment of the disease in an early stage, almost to guarantee freedom from acute attacks of arthritis. Before effective treatment was available some gouty patients used to die eventually of kidney failure caused by the deposition of uric acid crystals in the ureters and kidney parenchyma. Treatment may be considered under the headings, treatment of the acute attack and treatment of chronic gout.

TREATMENT OF THE ACUTE ATTACK

It is now known that the acute attack of gout develops because uric acid crystals form in the joint and irritate the polymorphonuclear leucocytes in the fluid within the joint. Pain develops when the polymorphs, having phagocytosed the uric acid crystals, die and liberate certain chemicals which cause the occurrence of intense inflammation. Colchicine has been the traditional remedy for acute gout for hundreds of years, but indomethacin and phenylbutazone are better.

Colchicine

Colchicine has a rather interesting mechanism of action in relieving the pain of an acute attack of gout. The drug prevents the polymorphonuclear leucocyte from ingesting further crystals of uric acid. The leucocyte is thus saved from an untimely death, it ceases to liberate chemicals which would induce further inflammation and the painful attack of gout accordingly improves.

Colchicine is usually given by mouth although it can on occasion be given intravenously if a rapid action is required.

It is common practice to give 1 mg orally and to instruct the patient to take 0.5 mg thereafter at two-hourly intervals until either relief of pain is experienced or diarrhoea occurs. Diarrhoea is the first side effect of colchicine and the drug *must* be stopped when this appears.

Colchicine can also be given as maintenance treatment to *prevent* acute attacks of gout. Doses of the order of 0.5 mg twice daily are used to do this.

Indomethacin and phenylbutazone

These drugs are discussed earlier. Both are used in high doses in acute gout and each starts to bring relief in an hour or so. There is nothing to choose between them as far as efficacy is concerned except that phenylbutazone carries with it a slight risk of inducing agranulocytosis. Indomethacin does not.

TREATMENT OF CHRONIC GOUT

When the blood uric acid is lowered to normal values (about 6.0 mg per cent in men and 5.0 mg per cent in women) there is much less risk of gouty patients developing an acute attack of gout. Uric acid is formed in the body in great amounts from certain foods notably liver, heart, kidneys, pancreas and brain.

Patients with severe chronic gout should be advised to abstain from these foods. A decrease in alcohol intake if it is normally high should also be advocated because alcohol prevents the elimination of uric acid from the body by the kidneys. A number of drugs are available which will reduce the uric acid level in the blood and so prevent attacks of gout and also prevent damage to the kidney. In the past drugs were used which increased the excretion of uric acid by kidneys, probenecid being the most popular. Unfortunately although this reduced the uric acid levels in the blood, it led to fairly high concentrations in the kidney and carried the risk of inducing kidney damage. Modern treatment reduces the formation of uric acid within the body.

Allopurinol

This agent lowers serum uric acid levels by preventing the formation of uric acid from its precursors in the body. Allopurinol is now the drug of first choice in the treatment of gout. It is especially valuable in treating gouty patients with renal insufficiency. You will often see allopurinal used along with cytotoxic drugs in the treatment of certain malignant diseases. This is because death of cell nuclei liberates large amount of uric acid precursors into the circulation. The levels of uric acid may rise to a great extent with resulting kidney damage.

An unusual fact is that allopurinol will sometimes induce an acute attack of gout in susceptible individuals soon after treatment is started. For this reason an anti-inflammatory drug such as indomethacin or colchicine is usually administered with allopurinol in the initial stages of treatment. It is possible to discontinue this later on.

9

Drugs acting on the haemopoietic system. Anticoagulants

This chapter describes drugs which are used in the treatment of anaemia and also the more commonly used anticoagulants.

ANAEMIA

Anaemia may be conveniently defined as a lack of circulating haemoglobin. Anaemia is measured therefore in terms of the haemoglobin which the blood contains. In men the normal haemoglobin concentration should be above 13 g per 100 ml of blood and in women this figure should be 12 g per 100 ml of blood. Values less than these may be said to be indicative of anaemia.

Causes of anaemia

All anaemias are caused basically in one of two ways or in a combination of these ways.

1. Premature loss or destruction of red blood cells
2. Incomplete replacement of red blood cells.

Acute or chronic loss of blood is an example of the first mechanism of causation of anaemia. A deficiency of iron or vitamin B12 or folic acid, all of which are necessary for the manufacture of haemoglobinated red cells in the bone marrow, provides an example of the second way in which anaemia may come about.

In iron deficiency anaemia the number of red cells produced by the bone marrow is normal but the concentration of haemoglobin in each cell is reduced. In pernicious anaemia inadequate numbers of cells are produced by the bone marrow but each cell contains a normal or an even increased concentration of haemoglobin. In either event the net effect is that the total concentration of circulating haemoglobin is reduced.

Iron

Iron is an essential element in the body, being vital for the production of haemoglobin, the muscle protein myoglobin, and certain important enzyme systems. A normal diet can contain more than the body's normal daily requirement for iron. Men lose very little iron in the urine, faeces and sweat. Usually the daily loss of iron equals the daily intake and it is unusual for men to become iron deficient unless they have a pathological condition leading to excessive blood loss, for instance a peptic ulcer. Because of blood loss during even a normal menstral period a woman's requirement for iron is approximately twice that of a man. As a result, even normal women of child-bearing age can become iron deficient. During pregnancy and lactation the demand for iron is even higher and iron supplements are routinely given to expectant and feeding mothers. Iron deficiency anaemia is thus common in women throughout the world, especially in those parts where pregnancy is frequent and the diet inadequate.

Apart from physiological causes in women, such as menstruation, pregnancy and lactation, iron deficiency anaemia has other causes in both sexes. These are:

1. Nutritional iron deficiency
2. Acute or chronic blood loss
3. Malabsorption of iron.

Nutritional iron deficiency

The foods rich in iron are meat, liver, eggs, spinach, dried fruit, nuts and chocolate, thus people with food fads and those who live alone and do not bother to prepare proper meals for themselves may become iron deficient. Elderly men who live alone are particularly at risk as many of them do not bother to cook meat or eggs and tend to live on bread, butter and tea. These foods are not rich in iron.

Acute or chronic blood loss

The most common cause of blood loss from the alimentary tract is gastric or duodenal ulceration. Gastric carcinoma, hiatus hernia, oesophageal varices and haemorrhoids can all cause loss of blood from the body. When red blood cells are lost they take with them their iron-containing haemoglobin content. In this way the patient becomes deficient in iron and less haemoglobin is incorporated in the new red blood cells.

Malabsorption of iron

Deficient absorption of iron from the intestine is a relatively rare cause of iron-deficiency anaemia. It may occur because the small intestinal mucosa is damaged or deficient as in celiac disease or Crohn's disease but more commonly malabsorption results from partial gastrectomy. Iron absorption is poor after partial gastrectomy because of deficient secretion of acid.

It is important that you understand that an attempt must be made to identify the precise cause in each case of iron deficiency anaemia. This is particularly important in elderly patients in whom anaemia may be the first sign of an occult tumour in the gastrointestinal tract. If the tumour is situated in the large bowel then early diagnosis and surgical treatment sometimes results in complete cure.

PREPARATIONS OF IRON

Iron can be given to patients orally, intramuscularly or intravenously. Therapy should be continued after the haemoglobin concentrations return to normal to replenish the body's stores of iron.

Ferrous sulphate

Ferrous sulphate is the simplest and the least expensive preparation of iron for oral administration and as such it is the drug of first choice. It is often given in a dose of one tablet (200 mg) three times a day. It is widely assumed that ferrous sulphate frequently leads to gastrointestinal upset. As most doctors and nurses and many patients expect this side effect then it is perhaps not surprising that many patients complain of problems once they have started therapy. In fact, true gastrointestinal disturbance doesn't happen very frequently and any patient with iron deficiency anaemia should be given a proper trial of ferrous sulphate before they are switched to any other preparation. If genuine problems do occur then some of the other drugs listed below can be used. The faeces of patients taking oral iron are coloured black and continued use sometimes causes a degree of constipation.

Ferrous fumarate

Each 200 mg tablet contains 65 mg of iron. These tablets are less likely to be mistaken for sweets by toddlers and young children. Death may result from the ingestion of even a few iron tablets in early childhood.

Sustained release preparations

Specially formulated preparations of iron are available which release the iron into the gastrointestinal tract over a period of hours. They are claimed to cause less gastric upset. In some cases they do seem to result in a genuine reduction in side effects. In general they only have to be given once daily but they are naturally more expensive and there is some doubt as to whether the amount of iron which is actually absorbed during treatment is as great as with the standard preparations.

Preparations of iron for parenteral administration

Oral iron therapy is so effective that it is rarely necessary to give iron intramuscularly or intravenously. You may be surprised to hear that the rise in haemoglobin following oral iron administration is just as fast as following parenteral administration. Parenteral iron therapy should therefore only be considered for those patients who have a genuine problem. Examples of this are true malabsorption of iron, true intolerance of orally administered iron and occasionally patients with severe anaemia in late pregnancy. The other indication of course is when a patient with iron deficiency anaemia is unreliable and regularly forgets to take treatment. Two preparations are available, iron dextran and iron sorbitol. Adverse reactions to iron dextran are fairly rare but intramuscular injection is painful, causing local staining of the buttock. Iron sorbitol is therefore preferred for intramuscular use. It is possible to calculate how much iron a patient needs to replenish his body stores and then to give daily injection until the total deficit has been corrected. Alternatively, the total calculated dose may be infused intravenously at a single visit. This method although convenient carries with it the danger of precipitating a severe systematic reaction. This method is contraindicated in any patient with a history of asthma or other forms of allergy. It is a wise precaution to give a small test dose of iron to check for the reaction 24 hours before giving a total dose infusion.

HYDROXYCOBALAMIN (VITAMIN B12) AND FOLIC ACID

Absorption of vitamin B12

Vitamin B12 is necessary for the manufacture of red cells in the bone marrow. It is widely distributed in many foods but the richest source is liver. In order for vitamin B12 to be absorbed it must first be acted upon by a substance secreted by the normal gastric mucosa. This substance is termed 'intrinsic factor'. After the vitamin has reacted with intrinsic factor it moves out of the stomach into the small bowel where it is absorbed in the distal part of the ileum. If the vitamin does not react with intrinsic factor, it is not absorbed.

Anaemias due to vitamin B12 deficiency

As you might expect from the description of the normal mechanism of absorption of vitamin B12 given above, there are many disease states which can interfere with this mechanism. Some of the commonest are:

1. Pernicious anaemia
2. Total gastrectomy
3. Malabsorption syndrome and other diseases involving the distal ileum
4. Blind loops of bowel.

Pernicious anaemia

This is the most common disease to cause severe deficiency of vitamin B12. In pernicious anaemia the gastric lining shows complete atrophy. Intrinsic factor is thus not secreted by the gastric parietal cells and there is failure of absorption of dietary vitamin B12.

Total gastrectomy

Total gastrectomy removes the gastric parietal cells and there is subsequent failure of intrinsic factor secretion. The consequent malabsorption of vitamin B12 may not become apparent until many years after gastrectomy. This is because the body stores of vitamin B12 in the liver are usually adequate to keep the patient going for some time. As most total gastrectomies are performed for carcinoma of the stomach, most of these patients do not live long enough for the effects of malabsorption of vitamin B12 to become clinically obvious. Some patients who have had a partial gastrectomy performed for gastric ulcer, develop atrophy of the lining of the remaining portion of the stomach. These patients are then liable to develop malabsorption of vitamin B12.

Malabsorption syndrome and other diseases involving the distal ileum

The failure to absorb vitamin B12 is just one of a number of difficulties in absorption of nutrients which is experienced by patients with the malabsorption syndrome. Other diseases, such as Crohn's disease, may occasionally produce vitamin B12 deficiency by interfering with its absorption, if the terminal portion of the ileum is severely involved.

Blind loops of bowel

This is a rare though interesting cause of vitamin B12 deficiency.

Sometimes after a surgical operation a loop of bowel is created through which the contents of the intestinal lumen do not flow. When this happens bacteria are very liable to colonise the blind loop and live there happily ever after as it were, without being disturbed by the flow of intestinal contents. Vitamin B12 is a necessary food for these bacteria and they utilise it from the blood stream. Vitamin B12 deficiency then may develop. This rare condition responds quite satisfactorily to antibiotic therapy. As the bacteria are killed the state of vitamin B12 deficiency is reversed.

Clinical effects of vitamin B12 deficiency

There are three main clinical effects of deficiency of this vitamin: atrophic glossitis, megaloblastic anaemia and subacute combined degeneration of the spinal cord. Fortunately in most patients the diagnosis is made before the last of these conditions supervenes. If the diagnosis of vitamin B12 deficiency is delayed, however, the condition of subacute combined degeneration of the cord can cause paralysis of the patient's legs. This is because vitamin B12 is necessary for the proper functioning of the nervous system.

The patient with atrophic glossitis complains of a smooth red painful tongue. This may be the first clue to the presence of vitamin B12 deficiency and may become obvious long before the onset of anaemia. The anaemia of vitamin B12 deficiency is megaloblastic. This means that not only is there a dearth of red blood cells in the blood but that the precursors of these red cells in the bone marrow have an abnormal form. These abnormal bone marrow precursors are referred to as megaloblasts.

Hydroxycobalamin

Pernicious anaemia, a condition which nearly always proved fatal in the past, can be treated most effectively with vitamin B12. Although patients will respond to massive doses of vitamin B12 administered orally such therapy is impractical and the drug in practice is always given by intramuscular injection. Two preparations are available, hydroxycobalamin and cyanocobalamin. Hydroxycobalamin is the best preparation and should be the one routinely used. A patient with pernicious anaemia usually receives daily injections of 1000 ug for one week and then continues to receive 1000 ug monthly for the rest of his or her life. It is essential that this fact is impressed upon the patient as discontinuation of therapy through lack of understanding can have disastrous results.

Folic acid

Folic acid is present in liver, yeast and green vegetables. Deficiency of folic acid may develop in a number of circumstances including poor dietary intake, disease of the small intestine leading to malabsorption, pregnancy, alcoholism, and is a side effect of phenytoin and the barbiturate drugs. As already mentioned, the body has extensive stores of vitamin B12 and deficiency takes several years to develop. By contrast the body does not store folic acid effectively and deficiency of folic acid with resulting anaemia can develop with remarkable rapidity under conditions of reduced intake or increased demand such as in pregnancy. The anaemia of folic acid deficiency is indistinguishable from that of vitamin B12 deficiency. The appearances of the red blood cells and the bone marrow are identical. Sensitive laboratory tests which measure the level of folic acid in the blood provide the diagnosis. Therapy with folic acid is very effective and unlike vitamin B12 this can be given orally, usually in a dose of between 5 and 20 mg per day.

ANTICOAGULANT THERAPY

Anticoagulants are drugs which interfere with the clotting properties of the blood. The most frequently used anticoagulants in clinical practice are heparin and the coumarin derivatives phenindione and warfarin.

Mechanism of normal blood coagulation

The mechanism whereby blood clots is an extremely complicated one and it is not yet fully understood. A great deal is, however, known about some of the factors which contribute to normal blood clotting. It is not necessary that you be familiar with the intricate details of this complex subject but it would probably be helpful if you understand a little about the processes which initiate the formation of a clot so that you may have a clearer grasp of how anticoagulant drugs act to produce their effect. A simplified mechanism of blood clotting is illustrated in Figure 9.1.

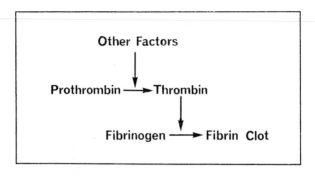

Fig. 9.1. A simplified diagram of blood clotting.

When a clot forms in the body it is composed of a vast number of extremely tiny strands of a protein called fibrin. These strands form a mesh which traps red blood cells in its lattices. Fibrin does not normally occur in the body. It is present as a soluble precursor, fibrinogen, which circulates in the blood stream. When a clot forms, soluble fibrinogen is converted to insoluble fibrin which lays down the lattice already referred to. The conversion of fibrinogen to fibrin is effected through the action of another component in the blood, thrombin. Unless thrombin is present in the circulation, fibrinogen will not be converted to fibrin. Thrombin itself is not normally present in the circulation but circulates as a precursor known as prothrombin. There are a large number of other factors needed in the blood stream to allow prothrombin to be converted to thrombin. If you cut your finger a great number of changes take place in the blood chemistry at the site of the cut. These changes eventually cause prothrombin to become thrombin; this in turn causes fibrinogen to become fibrin, and a clot is formed.

Anticoagulant drugs exert their effect by depressing the formation or the action of one or other of the blood coagulation factors.

Heparin

This is prepared from the mast cells in the lungs of cattle. Mast cells are full of granules particularly rich in heparin. The drug acts by inhibiting the conversion of fibrinogen to fibrin by antagonising the effect of thrombin. It has a very rapid onset of action.

Heparin can be given by intramuscular injection but has the disadvantage of being liable to produce a large haemorrhage in the muscle at the site of the injection. Even small haemorrhages in muscle are extremely painful and for this reason heparin should be given intravenously rather than intramuscularly.

Heparin may be given either by regular bolus intravenous injection, say 4 to 6-hourly, or by continuous intravenous infusion delivered through a standard drip and giving set or a constant infusion pump. Heparin is usually given when there is an urgent need to reduce the coagulability of the blood. The commonest indication is when a patient has developed a deep vein thrombosis of the leg or part of this clot has broken off and produced a pulmonary embolus. Sometimes heparin is given because the patient appears to be at particular risk of developing a deep vein thrombosis. A common example of this is following a myocardial infarction. It is important that you realise that heparin does not accelerate the breakdown of blood clot but merely prevents further development of fresh thrombus from this which is more liable to lead to embolisation. The dose of heparin required to anticoagulate the patient varies. An average dose is 20 000 units given intravenously over 12 hours. If the patient is elderly or very thin, then the dose may have to be reduced otherwise excessive anticoagulation and bleeding will result. Heparin is usually given for the first 48 hours of anticoagulant therapy. At the end of this period orally administered anticoagulants such as phenindione or warfarin have usually had time to take their effect and treatment with heparin may then be stopped. Occasionally heparin is given by intravenous infusion for periods of up to 10 days but side effects seem to be more common with this form of therapy. Naturally the main adverse effect of heparin is tendency to haemorrhage and patients with a possible bleeding site, for instance a peptic ulcer or an increased tendency to cerebral haemorrhage, for instance in hypertension, are greatly at risk. These patients should not receive heparin unless the benefit greatly outweighs the risk. If too much heparin is given and an antidote is necessary, protamine sulphate is given intravenously.

'Low dose' heparin

In recent years it has been discovered that low doses of heparin, for instance 5000 units every 8 hours, giver subcutaneously prevent the development of deep vein thrombosis in patients with an increased tendency to clotting, for instance after hip surgery. This form of therapy seems very safe in that the doses used don't lead to an increased tendency to haemorrhage. Heparin when given by this route seems to act in a different fashion from when it is given in full doses. This form of therapy is not effective in a patient who has already developed deep vein thrombosis or pulmonary embolus.

Fibrinolytic agents

These are not strictly anticoagulant drugs as they do not directly affect blood clotting. Instead they actively break down and dissolve the fibrin network which is the basis of a blood clot. Streptokinase is the drug most commonly used and this is given by constant intravenous infusion when massive pulmonary embolism has occurred. With less severe cases of embolism conventional anticoagulants are used. Fibrinolytic agents are dangerous and frequently lead to sensitivity reactions. Hydro-cortisone is usually given to prevent this.

Coumarin derivatives (warfarin and phenindione)

The coumarin anticoagulants were discovered in an interesting way. It was noticed some years ago that a herd of cattle had developed a severe bleeding tendency. The cause of this new disease was traced to a crop of over-ripe clover which these cattle had been eating. Further research into this clover pro-duced the coumarin anticoagulants. These drugs act principally by suppressing the formation of prothrombin by the liver (Fig. 9.1). It is not until 48 hours or so after their administration that the level of prothrombin in the blood becomes sufficiently reduced for an anticoagulant effect to be seen.

The principle of administration of these drugs is fairly similar to that which underlies the administration of digoxin (Ch. 3). A loading dose of the anticoagulant drug is followed by a small maintenance dose to suit the individual needs of the patient. Phenindione has a slightly shorter duration of action than warfarin and is given twice daily. Warfarin is given once daily. The amount of anticoagulant drug which each patient requires is assessed by making indirect measurements of the concentration of prothrombin in the blood. This may be either the prothrombin time or the thrombotest. The thrombotest is a more rapid assessment of the anticoagulant effect and is used widely to adjust the maintenance dose of anticoagulant each patient needs. In practice, warfarin is used more commonly than phenindione as the latter is more likely to cause toxicity, particularly skin rashes. The required dose of warfarin tends to vary from patient to patient but usually lies in the range 3 to 8 mg per day. Patients on long-term anticoagulant therapy need to attend hospital regularly for a thrombotest. If the thrombotest is outwith the desired range then the dose of warfarin may have to be adjusted up or down. This ensures an adequate state of anticoagulation and also prevents haemorrhage due to the excessive anticoagulation.

Indications for anticoagulant therapy

Anticoagulant therapy may be given for either a short period (6 weeks to 6 months,) or long-term. Sometimes this means lifelong therapy.

Short-term therapy

Patients who sustain deep vein thrombosis of the legs with or without a pulmonary embolus generally receive anticoagulants with the aim of preventing further clotting. These patients may have a condition predisposing them to pathological clotting such as recent surgery or use of a contraceptive pill. In the latter example an episode of thrombosis is an absolute contraindication to further use of the contraceptive pill as further thrombosis, possibly with massive embolisation, may occur. When the risk of further thrombosis seems to be passed, then anticoagulants can be stopped. There are no hard and fast rules but most patients are kept on warfarin for at least 2 months following an episode of thrombosis. Anticoagulant drugs have not been shown to have any benefit in preventing thrombosis in the coronary arteries although sometimes they are given to patients following a myocardial infarction to prevent thrombosis in the deep veins of the legs.

Long-term therapy

Anticoagulant drugs have to be given indefinitely to patients who have stenosis of the mitral valve and an irregular cardiac rhythm (atrial fibrillation). This is because thrombosis tends to develop in the left atrium and may cause embolisation into the major arteries of the body. Patients who have had a prosthetic heart valve may also be at risk and anticoagulant drugs help to prevent small thrombi developing on the heart valve itself. Occasionally patients who have recurrent venous thrombosis for which an underlying cause has not been found or treated, are left on long-term anticoagulant therapy. In all these instances the drug of choice is warfarin.

Contraindications to anticoagulant therapy

It is obvious that patients who have a possible bleeding source, for instance a peptic ulcer or ulcerative colitis, may develop massive haemorrhage if they are anticoagulated. In many patients, therefore, these conditions contraindicate the use of anticoagulant drugs. In some cases, however, the patient may be at risk of dying from a pulmonary embolus and a difficult decision then has to be made about anticoagulant therapy. Nowadays an attempt will be made to assess the activity of a peptic ulcer for instance by gastroscopy, or the degree of inflammation of the colon by sigmoidoscopy, and if the risk does not seem too great then the patient may be carefully anticoagulated. Other groups of patients seem particulary at risk of haemorrhage. This includes old people, and here the decision to anticoagulate has to be made very carefully. Patients with hypertension of any severity are at risk of a cerebral haemorrhage and this will often be regarded as a complete contraindication to drugs like warfarin. Patients with severe liver disease in general should not receive anticoagulants. In liver disease there is a diminished level of prothrombin in the blood because this substance is normally synthesised in the liver. Patients with renal disease are also very sensitive to anticoagulants. In both of these conditions it is therefore very difficult to control anticoagulant therapy satisfactorily.

There are many drugs which interfere with anticoagulants. Certain of these drugs, for instance phenylbutazone, aspirin and clofibrate increase the tendency to haemorrhage by displacing the warfarin from the protein it is bound to within the blood. Careless use of one of these drugs, therefore, may lead to serious haemorrhage. Some antibiotics kill off certain bacteria in the gut which make vitamin K. Vitamin K is an antidote to coumarin anticoagulants (see below) and the reduced levels lead to increased risk of haemorrhage. Phenytoin, barbiturates and a few other drugs increase the activity of the enzymes in the liver responsible for the breakdown of coumarin anticoagulants. If these drugs are therefore started, the levels of drug in the blood and the liver fall quickly and as a result the patient becomes less anticoagulated. If these drugs are used, therefore, the dose of anticoagulant drug may have to be increased to keep the patient in the therapeutic range. It is a good rule to tell your patient on an anticoagulant never to take any compound without first consulting a doctor, even simple cold 'cures' bought in a grocer's shop may contain aspirin or some other drug which seriously interferes with anticoagulant therapy and this may produce the risk of serious haemorrhage. (See also Ch. 13).

Side effect of coumarin derivatives

Obviously the main side effect of these drugs is haemorrhage. Haemorrhage may occur in anybody whose prothrombin level in the blood has been reduced too far by excessive anticoagulant therapy. Haemorrhage may occur from the gastrointestinal tract, causing haematemesis and melaena, or the urinary tract resulting in haematuria. Occasionally, cerebral haemorrhage occurs and this is disastrous. With proper anticoagulant control, however, this should not happen, and in fact serious haemorrhage is relatively rare considering the number of patients who receive anticoagulant drugs. Clearly, patients who have a possible bleeding site may haemorrhage despite proper anticoagulant control and the answer here is careful selection of patients for therapy. Occasionally skin rashes and drug fever occur and this happens more commonly with phenindione. This drug often gives a pink colour to the urine which is mistaken for blood. It is worthwhile warning your patient about this in case he or she becomes alarmed.

Antidote to the coumarins

It is more difficult to reverse the effect of coumarin anticoagulants than it is to reverse the effects of heparin. Warfarin and phenindione reduce the activity of vitamin K within the liver. Their anticoagulant effect therefore can be counteracted by giving large doses of vitamin K intravenously. Full correction of the deficiency, however, may take 24 hours or more as the effects of these drugs, and in particular warfarin, are delayed. In severe cases of haemorrhage, blood clotting factors may be given to the patient, either as the specific concentrate of the clotting factor or in the form of fresh frozen plasma. This is rarely necessary.

10

Drugs used in the treatment of malignant disease

The treatment of cancer traditionally has three arms: surgery, radiotherapy and drugs, used individually or in combination. In some diseases, for instance leukaemia, drugs offer the best treatment. More commonly they are used in addition to surgery or radiotherapy (adjuvant treatment). Sometimes they are used because other treatment has failed. Tumour cells differ from normal cells in that they exhibit uncontrolled growth, and cytotoxic drugs are designed to exploit this difference. A drug that selectively destroys tumour cells but does little or no damage to normal cells has not yet been discovered. Anticancer drugs currently available act on malignant cells by damaging biochemical pathways that are also present in normal cells. It is therefore not surprising that the therapeutic dose of these drugs is very close to the toxic dose and the risk of killing rather than curing is a major factor restricting the use of these drugs. Because rapidly dividing cells are most readily affected, damage occurs particularly in the bone marrow and intestinal mucosa. This may cause anaemia, a low white count with the risk of infection (agranulocytosis) or a low platelet count with the risk of bleeding (thrombocytopenia). The effects in the gut commonly include vomiting and diarrhoea as well as ulceration of the mouth (gingivitis). Another major complication is the suppression of the normal response to infection with reduction in antibody formation, as well as the depression of the white cell count. Because of these effects infection may be a life-threatening complication of treatment. Less serious, but disturbing to the patient, is alopecia (baldness) due to suppression of hair growth.

Because of these problems patients receiving intensive drug therapy are often nursed in special units where extra precautions are taken to protect them against infection. Supportive treatment may be given for bone marrow suppression with blood and platelet transfusion for anaemia and bleeding and occasionally white cell transfusion for infection. Intensive antibiotic treatment may be necessary. Where drugs are used to cure the disease a higher level of toxicity is acceptable than if drugs are merely being used as palliation, i.e. to relieve symptoms but without hope of permanent cure.

Drugs may be used alone or in combination with other agents. When a number of drugs are used in combination each drug should have a different mode of action and should if possible produce different forms of toxicity. As in multiple chemotherapy in tuberculosis (see Ch. 5) cytotoxic drugs in combination reduce the risk of drug resistance developing and increase the chance of tumour suppression.

CLASSES OF DRUGS IN COMMON USE

Cytotoxic drugs fall into four main groups.

1. Alkylating agents

These have an effect similar to that of X-rays on tumour tissue, causing structural damage to chromosomes.

Cyclophosphamide

Is one of the most commonly used. Its principle adverse reaction is baldness, which is reversible, and nausea and vomiting to which tolerance develops. It may occasionally produce an inflammation of the bladder, called haemorrhagic cystitis, which is very distressing to the patient. It is rapidly absorbed orally and may also be given intravenously. It is used mainly in the treatment of lymphomas (tumours of lymphoid tissue) and may be effective in chemotherapy of solid tumours such as breast cancer.

Mustine

Mustine is given intravenously and the major problem associated with its use is inflammation of the vein at the site of injection. Severe ulceration of the tissue may occur if the drug leaks out of the vein. For this reason it is usually injected slowly into a fast-running, well-sited intravenous infusion. It is used most frequently in the treatment of Hodgkin's disease (a common form of lymphoma).

Thiotepa

This drug may be given into the peritoneum in the treatment of malignant ascites. It is not as commonly used as some of the other agents mentioned.

Busulphan and chlorambucil

These are useful drugs which are given orally in the management of chronic leukaemias. They are not as toxic as some of the other agents mentioned in this section and are usually given over much longer periods. As the prognosis in chronic leukaemia is very much better than in many other malignant diseases it is important that the treatment given does not produce unacceptable toxicity. Bone marrow depression may develop during the course of treatment with either of these drugs but it is more serious when it occurs in association with busulphan as it may be irreversible.

2. Antimetabolites

These drugs act by damaging a vital part of the internal chemistry of the tumour cell, so preventing its growth and replication.

Folic acid antagonists

Methotrexate is very similar in structure to folic acid and prevents the action of folic acid by competitive inhibition This will prevent growth of cancer cells and also other rapidly dividing tissue such as bone marrow and intestinal mucosa. The principle side effects of methotrexate therefore are bone marrow suppression, diarrhoea and oral ulceration. When the drug is used in high doses some of these effects may be reversed by giving folinic acid which bypasses the essential stage in nucleic acid synthesis which is blocked by methotrexate. Methotrexate occasionally leads to damage of the lungs and when used over long periods liver damage has resulted. It is usually given intravenously but may also be given orally or intrathecally. It is widely used in the treatment of leukaemia and as adjuvant therapy in the treatment of solid tumours such as breast cancer. It has proved very successful in the management of the trophoblastic tumour chorion-carcinoma.

Antipurines and antipyrimidines

These interfere with the incorporation of the essential compounds, purine and pyrimidine into the nucleic acids thus stopping the formation of chromosomes.

6Mercaptopurine. This is used in the treatment of acute leukaemia. In addition to the usual side effects in the bone marrow, it may cause jaundice.

5 Fluorouracil. This drug is given intravenously and is used in the treatment of tumours of the gastrointestinal tract, the breast and gynaecological growths.

Cytosine arabinoside. Is given intravenously and acts mainly on the bone marrow. It is therefore used in the treatment of acute leukaemia.

3. Spindle poisons

These prevent the normal division of chromosomes during mitosis. The most important are vincristine and vinblastine. These drugs cause little bone marrow suppression but may result in damage to nerves, giving rise to pain, and weakness. They are given intravenously in acute leukaemias and Hodgkin's disease.

4. Antibiotics

Like the antibiotic drugs used for the treatment of infection (Ch.

5), these drugs are derived from living organisms. Many were first developed for the treatment of infection but they are much too toxic for this indication and their use is confined to the treatment of malignant disease.

Actinomycin D

This is used in conjunction with radiation in childhood tumours and may be used in tumours of ovary and testis in adults. It is given intravenously and like mustine is highly irritant if it leaks from the vein.

Daunorubicin

This drug is very useful given intravenously in acute leukaemia in adults. In addition to the usual side effects of cytotoxic drugs it has a specific toxic action on heart muscle. This restricts the total dose which may be used.

Adriamycin

This drug is given intravenously in acute leukaemias and some solid tumours.

Corticosteroids

Corticosteroids are very widely used in the drug treatment of malignant disease. Their action in this situation is complex. They seem to suppress lymphoid tissue making them useful in the treatment of lymphoid tumours and lymphatic leukaemia. They also tend to increase the neutrophil and platelet count in the blood, making them valuable in the treatment of patients with marrow depression. In addition to these actions they reduce swelling and inflammation in tissues and also produce a feeling of wellbeing in the patient. The actions and side effects of corticosteroids are discussed in detail in Chapter 8.

Uses of cytotoxic drugs

Leukaemias

Leukaemia is a malignant proliferation of abnormal white blood cells. In childhood the most common form is acute lymphatic leukaemia in which cytotoxic therapy has been so successful that some patients may now be described as cured. Treatment of patients with leukaemia involves two stages, the first stage is to induce a remission. A remission means that the white cell count in the blood has been returned to normal and the clinical features of the disease have regressed. This is usually achieved with a combination of vincristine and prednisolone. The second stage is maintenance therapy in which the original remission is prolonged by using methotrexate and 6 mercaptopurine. This is given for at least 2 years. Recurrence of disease within the central nervous system is prevented by radiation. This leads to total baldness. Acute leukaemia in adults is much more difficult to treat and few are cured. The same principle of inducing a remission followed by maintenance therapy is used. Several drugs in combination may be necessary for the first stage and this commonly produces severe toxicity. A wide variety of drugs is used in various combinations and it is not possible to cover these in detail.

Chronic leukaemia is an adult disease and the outlook is very much better than in acute leukaemia. For this reason, treatment is much less intensive and less toxicity results. Chlorambucil, busulphan and cyclophosphamide are commonly used. In this condition single drugs rather than combination have proved successful. Patients with chronic leukaemia may survive for many years and in some no treatment is necessary.

Lymphomas

These are cancers of the lymphoid tissue. They fall into two groups. Hodgkin's disease is the commonest, the other group is now known as non-Hodgkin's lymphomas. Many patients with Hodgkin's disease can be be cured by the correct treatment. As different treatment has to be given for different stages of the disease, intensive investigation is initially carried out. Local disease confined to one area is usually treated by radiotherapy. More extensive disease requires chemotherapy. Several drugs are usually used in combination and the most popular regime is **Mustine**, vincristine (called **O**ncovin), **P**rednisolone and **P**rocarbazine. For obvious reasons this drug regimen is known as MOPP. A course of treatment lasts 2 weeks and this is always followed by a two week rest period. At least six courses of treatment are usually given and in some cases treatment may be continued for a year or more. The treatment of non-Hodgkin's lymphomas has followed the same lines but has not been nearly so successful. The drugs used include cyclophosphamide, vincristine and prednisolone.

Solid tumours

Some solid tumours in childhood which are derived from embryonic tissues are very sensitive to cytotoxic drugs, and cure has been achieved in Wilms' tumour of the kidney by using actinomycin D in addition to surgery and radiotherapy. In adults the use of drugs has been much less successful and drug treatment in general has a limited role. In breast cancer, surgery may be followed by either radiotherapy with hormonal drugs or use of some of the agents mentioned above. The drugs commonly used are cyclophosphamide, methotrexate and 5 fluorouracil. In tumours of the gastrointestinal tract, genitourinary system, head, neck and brain, drugs may be used in treatment of the advanced stages but in general success is very limited.

Only in the rare tumour, chorioncarcinoma, derived from the placenta, have the results been satisfactory. Many women suffering from this tumour have been cured by the drug methotrexate.

11

Drugs used in Disorders of the Endocrine System

This chapter deals with drugs used in the treatment of diabetes mellitus and discusses the treatment of some disorders of the thyroid, adrenal and pituitary glands. A brief review of the uses and actions of the male and female sex hormones is also included together with a discussion of the mode of action of the contraceptive pill. As diabetes mellitus is the commonest endocrine disorder and as it is essential that you have a clear knowledge of the uses of insulin in its treatment, most of this chapter will deal with this hormone.

DIABETES MELLITUS

This is a condition in which the islets of Langerhans in the pancreas fail to secrete enough insulin to meet the requirements of the body. As a result the blood glucose becomes elevated and some of the excess glucose is excreted in the urine. There are, broadly speaking, two sorts of patients with diabetes mellitus. The first is typically a young thin subject who tends to develop diabetes early in life. He has a tendency to develop diabetic coma and the state of his diabetes is sensitive to insulin treatment. The second sort of patient is typically a middle-aged obese woman who develops diabetes in later life. She does not have the same liability to develop diabetic coma as the first kind of patient and her disease tends to be resistant to insulin treatment, but is controlled satisfactorily with diet and oral hypoglycaemic agents. This division is a slight simplification of the true state of affairs but is, generally speaking, true. In general, therefore, younger patients tend to require insulin and older patients can be managed either by diet or by diet and drugs. There are of course occasional exceptions to this rule and sometimes it is necessary to give an elderly patient insulin if they cannot be managed by other means. It is unusual for a young person to be controlled satisfactorily on drugs.

Actions of insulin

You will use insulin a great deal in your professional life and it is therefore fitting that you should have some knowledge of how this substance acts to lower the blood glucose.

Insulin is secreted directly into the blood by the b cells of the islets of Langerhans in the pancreas. It may therefore be called a hormone. Insulin allows the entry of glucose into the cells of the body thereby facilitating its metabolism. When glucose is introduced into a cell under the action of insulin the electrolyte potassium is also taken into that cell along with glucose. This fact has a bearing on the clinical management of patients in diabetic coma being treated with insulin, as is discussed later.

Preparations of insulin

All insulin preparations have to be given by injection as the hormone is rapidly inactivated by enzymes in the stomach and jejunum if administered orally. Usually insulin is given by subcutaneous injection which is a relatively simple technique. The great majority of patients are trained to give themselves their own insulin. Human insulin is not available and the drug is therefore extracted from the pancreatic glands of cattle and pigs. Beef insulin was the form most widely used in the past but pork insulin has a similar structure to the human hormone and is becoming more popular. Standard beef insulins contain a number of impurities which tend to stimulate an antibody response by the body. Research in recent years has produced highly purified forms of porcine insulin sometimes called monocomponent insulins (see section on highly purified insulins). The aim of treatment in patients requiring insulin is to keep the blood sugar as near normal as possible throughout the 24 hours. When considering the type of insulin used, therefore, thought must be given to the length of its action. The time of onset of effect after injection, the time of maximum effect and total duration of effect are all important. Soluble insulin, for instance, has an onset of action within an hour of injection, a peak effect round 3 to 6 hours and a total duration of effect of less than 10 hours. Its highly purified pork equivalent, Actrapid, has an even shorter action (Table 11.1). Clearly a single injection of either of these preparations will not control diabetes throughout 24 hours. It is possible to alter the duration of action of insulin by combining it with the protein molecule protamine or a heavy metal (usually zinc) or both. This can be done either with the standard beef insulin or the highly purified porcine type. Modifying the insulin in this way means that it is released more slowly from the injection site in the subcutaneous tissues and wide variations in the time of action can be achieved (Table 11.1).

Principles of treatment of diabetics requiring insulin

Treatment of diabetic coma

Diabetic coma is also known as diabetic ketoacidosis. This is a grave medical emergency which in the past carried a high mortality. Death is now uncommon if effective treatment is started quickly. Diabetic coma may develop in any patient who is receiving insulin. Occasionally a previously undiagnosed diabetic will present in this fashion. Diabetic coma in a previously well-controlled diabetic may result from inadequate insulin dosage or because of infection, which reduces the effectiveness of insulin, and results in the patient becoming resistant to the normal dose of insulin. Sometimes no clear cut cause can be discovered. The features of diabetic coma, therefore, are brought about by lack of insulin. They are:

1. Hyperglycaemia (high blood sugar)
2. Acidosis
3. Dehydration.

Hyperglycaemia. When insulin is deficient glucose is unable to enter the body cells. The blood sugar is therefore very high and the cells must use another energy source for metabo-

Table 11.1 Characteristics of insulins in common use

Name	Type	Modification	Purity	Action	Time of action (Hrs after injection) Peak	Duration
Soluble	Beef	None	Standard	Short	3–6	10
Actrapid	Pork	None	Highly purified	Short	2–5	7
Semilente	Beef	IZS.†	Standard	Medium	3–8	16
Semitard	Pork	IZS †	Highly purified	Medium	4–9	16
Monotard	Pork	IZS †·	Highly purified	Medium	6–14	22
Isophane	Beef	Protamine	Standard	Medium/long	6–14	24
Retard	Pork	Protamine	Highly purified	Medium/long	4–12	24
Lente	Beef	IZS (Mixture)‡	Standard	Long	5–13	30
PZI	Beef	Protamine zinc insulin	Standard	Long	10–22	36

† IZS: insulin zinc suspension

‡ IZS: (mixture): mixture of medium and long acting forms of IZS designed to give a quick onset plus long duration of effect

lism. Treatment of hyperglycaemia is with short-acting insulins, either soluble insulin or Actrapid (Table 11.1). Insulin must *not* be given subcutaneously as it is not absorbed from this site in diabetic coma. It may be given either intravenously or by deep intramuscular injection. In the past very high bolus injections, for instance 100 units intravenously, were given in the treatment of diabetic coma. More recently, it has been discovered that treatment with low doses can be just as effective. If insulin is given in small doses intravenously in diabetic coma it must be by continuous infusion. This is because it disappears very quickly from the blood after a single injection and will only be effective for a short time. Modern regimens use infusion pumps to deliver doses of 4 to 12 units per hour. Insulin is absorbed more slowly after intramuscular injection, so that a dose of say 10 units given intramuscularly every hour is effective treatment of diabetic coma.

Acidosis. The deficiency of alkali arises in a rather curious fashion. Normally glucose is metabolised by the body to provide energy. In diabetic coma, glucose can no longer be metabolised and is therefore no longer available as a source of energy. The body deals with this situation by metabolising its fat stores in order to obtain the energy which it needs. The end products of the metabolism of fat are the substances acetone, hydroxybutyric acid and acetoacetic acid. The last two of these compounds are acids (*ketoacids,* hence the term ketoacidosis), and the body has to neutralize them with its reserves of alkali. As time goes on and the production of these acids increases, the deficiency of alkali (sodium bicarbonate) becomes very marked and the acid content of the blood increases. This becomes clinically obvious in three ways: the patient's respiratory centre is stimulated by excess acid in the blood, the breath reeks of acetone which smells like nail-varnish remover (acetone is the main ingredient of nail-varnish remover), and the urine becomes loaded with the two ketoacids and with acetone. These three substances are collectively referred to as ketones or ketone bodies.

Treatment of acidosis is usually very straightforward. Correction of the severe dehydration and administration of insulin results in very rapid correction of the blood pH level in the great majority of patients. The administration of sodium bicarbonate intravenously therefore is not usually necessary. In some cases, however, when the patient is very shocked, the acidosis can be so severe that life is threatened and in these cases sodium bicarbonate may have to be given. This is always done fairly carefully as the rapid correction of acidosis with alkaline solutions is not without risk and the level of potassium in the blood tends to fall precipitously.

Dehydration. Treatment of the severe dehydration of diabetic coma is just as important as administration of insulin. When the blood sugar is very high, it exceeds the renal threshhold for glucose and spills over in large quantities into the urine. When glucose is present in the urine it pulls water into the tubules by osmotic action. Vast quantities of fluid can be lost in this way and result in the common symptoms of uncontrolled diabetes — extreme thirst and polyuria. It is a common mistake to underestimate the deficiency of fluid which may be 6 litres or more. This deficiency is corrected with 0.9 per cent saline (see C. 12). It is vital that an accurate record of the fluid balance of the patient is kept. The amount of fluid infused must be checked against the volume of fluid excreted by the kidneys. Without accurate knowledge of the balance of input and output it is impossible to plan future fluid administration. The rate at which fluid is infused is often very high and in severe cases of diabetic coma more than 2 litres of saline may be administered within the first hour. Shortly after treatment is started with fluid and insulin, potassium enters the cells from the blood stream and the level in the plasma may fall very quickly. All diabetics therefore will require potassium chloride added to the infusion fluid. This is not usually administered in the first hour or two during which saline is being given very quickly, but thereafter large amounts of potassium are usually required (see potassium therapy pp 244-245).

Once the severe deficiencies noted above have been corrected an attempt is made to estimate how much insulin the patient will need in the future to control his diabetes. The amount of insulin administered during the treatment of diabetic coma is no guide. If the patient has been previously well controlled on a fixed regime, then that may simply be re-started after a stable condition has been achieved. If the patient is a new diabetic the condition may be controlled by injection of a short-acting insulin (soluble or Actrapid) three or four times daily before meals. The dose can be judged by a urine test performed shortly before the injection. This method of determining insulin dosage by the content of glucose in the urine is known as a 'sliding scale'. An example of a commonly used sliding scale is given in Table 11.2. With the availability of devices for rapid measurement of the blood sugar by the bed side it is likely that 'sliding scale' regimes, by which the dose of insulin is determined by the blood sugar rather than a urine test, will become popular.

It is frequently forgotten that when a continuous intravenous infusion of insulin is stopped after correction of the ketoacidosis insulin disappears from the blood within minutes. This means that unless a subcutaneous dose of insulin is administered shortly after stopping the infusion the blood sugar may start to rise very quickly.

Once the insulin requirement has been estimated the patient can be transferred to a maintenance regime and taught the technique of self-injection.

Table 11.2 Typical sliding scale for insulin dosage (usually given 6-hourly)

Urine test (% glucose)	Insulin dosage (soluble)
2	24 units
1	16 units
¼–½	12 units
0	8 units

Maintenance treatment with insulin

Once a patient has been started on insulin he will generally require it for the rest of his life. The aim of treatment is to keep the blood sugar levels as near normal as possible in order to prevent diabetic coma and also in the hope that this will prevent or delay the onset of diabetic complications. Table 11.1 lists a number of the insulin preparations in common use. A complete list would be most confusing. Individual preference amongst physicians for different combinations of insulin is very variable. It is not possible for you to learn all of them. There is no 'best combination'. Diabetics are usually controlled by once or twice daily injections of insulin.

Once daily injections. It would be most convenient if the blood sugar could be well controlled in every diabetic following a single dose of insulin injected every morning. You will remember from what was said earlier that simple insulins, for instance soluble or Actrapid are very effective but have a short duration of action. This means that they have to be given several times each day to keep the blood sugar under control. The addition of zinc or protamine increases the duration but also delays the onset of action so that a single dose of say protamine zinc insulin will not have any effect in the early part of the day. A combination of soluble insulin and protamine zinc insulin will provide reasonable control throughout 24 hours and this is a justifiably popular regime. You should note these two insulins should not be mixed in the same syringe as some of the soluble insulin will be converted to PZI. In practice they are usually given from two syringes into the same needle, rotating the needle through 180° between injections to avoid mixing the tissues. Another popular preparation is Lente. Although this is a single preparation it is in fact a mixture of two forms of insulin zinc suspension (amorphous and crystalline). One has a medium action the other (crystalline) is long acting and together they give reasonable control, in a proportion of diabetics, throughout 24 hours. This is a most convenient preparation to use as only a single injection is needed and it is simpler than soluble and PZI.

Unfortunately only a few diabetics can be really well controlled with Lente. A number of other insulins or combinations of insulins can provide control throughout 24 hours following a single injection but it is not necessary for you to remember them all. Soluble and PZI and Lente are still the most widely used.

In general, single injections are only effective when the patient requires modest doses of insulin, in practice up to 60 units per day in total. Use of single injections therefore is most common in children and in the occasional middle-aged or elderly diabetic who requires insulin. Insulin requirements increase quite sharply at puberty and the majority of insulin dependent diabetics are in their teens or twenties. They frequently need more than 60 units of insulin each day. It is not possible to achieve satisfactory control in many of these young diabetics with a single injection and it is wrong to continue such a regime merely for the sake of convenience. These patients are best controlled on twice daily injections of insulin.

Twice daily regimes. Because of their short action soluble or Actrapid insulin given twice daily may not provide adequate control throughout 24 hours, and thrice daily injections would be very inconvenient for most diabetics. For this reason most modern regimes incorporate a short and medium acting insulin mixed together and injected twice daily, usually before breakfast and before the evening meal. The short-acting insulin copes with the carbohydrate in the meal and the medium-acting preparation helps to 'smooth out' the blood sugar throughout the remainder of the day. By careful alteration of dosage very precise control may be achieved in many cases. The most popular regime is a combination of soluble and isophane insulin given before breakfast and before dinner. Unlike soluble and PZI these two insulins may be mixed safely in the same syringe. Other regimes are available and are becoming more popular. You will note from Table 11.1 that three of the highly purified insulins have a medium action — Semitard, Monotard and Retard — although they vary a bit in their duration of action, any one of them can be used with Actrapid in an identical fashion to soluble and isophane i.e. mixed in the same syringe and injected twice daily before the main meals. It is likely that in the future an increasing number of new diabetics will be commenced on such a combination.

Highly purified insulins. Until now highly purified insulins have been considered along with the older non-purified varieties. This is quite correct as use of the different types is virtually identical. It is becoming common for young diabetics to be started on a highly purified form at the time their condition is first diagnosed, in the hope that this will result in better control and fewer complications. It will be many years before this theory can be properly tested and there is no reason why the older varieties should not continue to be widely used meanwhile.

At present there are a number of situations in which a highly purified insulin is specifically indicated. They are as follows:

1. Generalised allergy to insulin. This is rare
2. Local reaction at the injection site. Sometimes the impurities in the standard beef insulin suspensions, for instance Lente or PZI result in local inflammation at the injection site. This may alter absorption from that area and a change to the equivalent highly purified form of insulin will usually solve the problem
3. Lipoatrophy. When conventional non-purified insulins are injected repeatedly into one area, for instance the lateral thigh, the fat layer of the subcutaneous tissues may become very thin. This is known as lipoatrophy and it results in indentations in the surface of the leg which are rather unattractive. It is a curious fact that a change to a highly purified

insulin will often restore the normal appearance of these areas if the insulin is injected into the affected site

4. Insulin resistance. A number of diabetics develop antibodies to the non-purified beef insulins and their total requirements may rise above 200 units per day. Changing to a highly purified insulin will often bring about a dramatic reduction in their requirement and an improvement in control of their diabetes. Since the change in dosage is abrupt and somewhat unpredictable such alterations are best carried out in hospital.

Instruction of diabetic patients in the technique of self injection

You will often be called upon to explain to a recently discovered diabetic the technique of self injection of insulin. If you work outside hospital you may often be asked by diabetic patients for advice in matters concerning the storage or handling of insulin.

All preparations of insulin should be kept in a cool place but should not be placed in a freezer. The drug should never be used after the expiry date quoted on the bottle. Patients should sterilise their syringes and needles frequently by boiling them in water for five minutes. These utensils can then be stored in spirit in a dish or in a syringe case. Figure 11.1 shows an insulin syringe. Each ml is graduated into 20 divisions and you should teach your patient to refer to these divisions as 'marks'.

Insulin preparations are available in three strengths in the United Kingdom: 20 units per ml; 40 units per ml and 80 units per ml. In practice the 20 strength is seldom used outside hospital. One *mark* on an insulin syringe will contain 1 *unit* of 20 strength or 2 *units* of 40 strength or 4 *units* of 80 strength. In other words a patient requiring 20 units of insulin would require 20 *marks* of 20 strength, 10 *marks* of 40 strength or 5 *marks* of 80 strength. Patients requiring large doses of insulin tend to use 80 strength to reduce the volume of the injection. This may seem perfectly straightforward but you will be surprised how often patients, medical and nursing staff all become hopelessly confused over the distinction between *marks* and *units*. Whenever a diabetic patient is being admitted to hospital for any reason it is essential that you establish exactly how much insulin they had been taking outside hospital and you must ensure that you know whether a patient is talking about 'marks' or 'units'.

Always instruct your patient to shake the insulin bottle before taking up the insulin for injection. He should do this because insulin zinc suspension tends to separate into two layers on standing, one containing insulin the other not. He should expel the spirit from his syringe and needle by moving the plunger of the syringe rapidly up and down and should then draw into the syringe a volume of air equivalent to the volume of fluid he is going to draw out of the bottle. After cleansing the top of the bottle with a little spirit, and introducing the needle through the rubber cap, he should inject air into the bottle. He will then be able to take the insulin up into his syringe quite easily.

The technique of subcutaneous injection has already been covered in Chapter 1. It is most important that diabetics regularly pull the plunger back before injecting insulin to ensure that the tip of the needle is not lodged in the small vein. Intravenous injection of insulin can result in rapid onset of hypoglycaemia. It is also most important that you ensure that the diabetic patient is injecting the insulin subcutaneously and not into the skin itself (intradermal injection). Intradermal injection is painful and absorption of insulin is altered.

Diabetic patients must learn to change their injections sites regularly and you should remind them that it is quite permissible for them to inject into the subcutaneous tissues of the abdominal wall. Many diabectics are curiously reluctant to use this site.

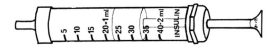

Fig.11.1. Diagram of an insulin syringe. The method of calculating units of insulin is explained in the text.

Hypoglycaemia (Low blood sugar)

Hypoglycaemia may result from any one of a number of possible causes. If a diabetic undertakes particularly vigorous physical activity, misses a meal or injects himself with too much insulin, the dangerous complication of hypoglycaemia may ensue. The patient may become quite suddenly confused and disorientated, he may become rude or aggressive or behave in a most peculiar way due to hypoglycaemia. If the condition is left untreated, unconsciousness and later death may ensue. All diabetic patients who are being controlled with insulin should carry on their person a card which proclaims them to be diabetic and the dose and preparation of insulin which they are receiving. The card should also state that if they are found unconscious or behaving in an odd fashion they should be given sugar-containing substances to eat and if this fails a doctor must be called immediately. You should check that your diabetic patient has such a card. If he does not he should be encouraged to obtain one from his own doctor.

Most diabetics who are receiving insulin experience some warning of the development of hypoglycaemia. This usually takes the form of sweating, a feeling of excessive hunger, shaking or nervousness. Once they have learned to recognise these early symptoms they can ward off the more serious effects of hypoglycaemia by taking something sweet. It is good practice to demonstrate the effects of mild hypoglycaemia to any new diabetic requiring insulin. This is done in hospital in a careful manner by withholding breakfast and administering an extra large dose of a short-acting insulin such as soluble or Actrapid. The effects when they develop can be quickly reversed. Unfortunately, some diabetics never seem to experience any real warning of the development of hypoglycaemia and these patients may become comatose before anybody realises that anything is wrong.

Diet in insulin-dependent diabetes

It is not possible in this short text to cover all the aspects of treatment of diabetes but a brief word on diet is necessary. Patients who receive a fixed dose of insulin each day must adhere to a diet which provides them with a fairly constant amount of carbohydrate. The total amount of carbohydrate consumed in 24 hours should be kept the same, as should the times at which it is taken. For this reason, insulin-dependent diabetics are given diets in which the total carbohydrate content is supplied in 10 g 'portions'. A diabetic might therefore be allocated 20 portions in 24 hours (200 g of carbohydrate). This could be given as five portions with each of the two main meals, four portions with breakfast and the remainder (six portions) in the form of milk and snacks distributed throughout the day. The distribution is fairly constant from day to day in any patient and depends partly on the type and dose of insulin being used. The total amount of carbohydrate is determined mainly by the nature of the patient's employment, a heavy labourer requiring a great deal more carbohydrate than an office worker. Although the amount and distribution of the carbohydrate intake remains constant, the type of food eaten can be varied and the diet made attractive by the use of 'exchanges'. With the knowledge of the carbohydrate content of any particular foodstuff a measured amount of this containing 10 g of carbohydrate can be exchanged for any other portion in the standard diet. All diabetics are supplied with a long list of exchanges which ensures that their diet varies from day to day. With most insulin-dependent diabetics it is only necessary to limit the carbohydrate content of their diet, their intake of protein and fats being unrestricted. The exception is the occasional patient who becomes obese necessitating a reduction in the calorific content of the diet. In this situation reduction of fat intake is necessary.

Treatment of diabetics who do not require insulin

Most diabetics who develop the condition in middle or old age can be satisfactorily treated without insulin. These patients tend not to develop severe ketoacidosis if left untreated, but they will experience disturbing symptoms in the form of thirst and polyuria due to glycosuria. Although their condition is milder than juvenile diabetics, some do long-term the serious long complications of the disease with resulting damage to the blood vessels, the eye and the kidney. In old age prevention of long-term complications is not a major consideration and treatment of diabetes aims to control the symptoms of thirst and polyuria and prevent dehydration.

In most of these 'mature onset' diabetics an attempt is first made to control the condition by diet alone. The type of diet used depends on the body weight. If the patient is obese a weight reduction diet, e.g. 1000 calories per day is prescribed. This of couse inevitably restricts their carbohydrate intake and if it is adhered to will dramatically reduce the symptoms of thirst and polyuria. If the patient successfully loses weight the diabetic tendency may disappear completely and the restrictions may then be relaxed. If the patient is thin or of normal weight the carbohydrate content of the diet is restricted, for instance 150 to 180 g per day. Free intake of protein and fat is allowed to ensure adequate calories. This often controls the condition, but in these patients it is sometimes necessary to prescibe a drug in order to lower the blood sugar. These drugs are known as oral hypoglycaemic agents. There are two groups of drugs — the sulphonylureas and the diguanides.

Sulphonylureas

This is a fairly large group of drugs with a similar structure to the sulphonamide antibacterial agents. They act by stimulating the pancreas to produce more insulin and are used in 'mature onset' diabetics whose condition has not been controlled by diet alone. Because they stimulate insulin release these drugs may lead to hypoglycaemia. Stimulation of the appetite results in weight gain. For this reason sulphonylureas should not routinely be given to overweight diabetics, although this is occasionally necessary if their condition is not adequately controlled by dieting. The most widely used drugs with typical dosages are:

Chlorpropamide: 100 to 500 mg per day
Tolbutamide: 500 to 2000 mg per day
Glibenclamide: 2.5 to 20 mg per day.

There are other members of this group. It is not necessary for you to remember all of them. The three drugs mentioned differ mainly in their duration of effect. Chlorpropamide acts for more than 30 hours and there is therefore a risk of accumulation, which is a particular hazard in the elderly who are very sensitive to the effects of hypoglycaemia. Glibenclamide is very potent but has a short action and is probably more suitable in old age.
Side effects are fairly uncommon with these drugs. Hypoglycaemia is an obvious risk which can be guarded against. A rash sometimes develops and jaundice is a rare complication with chlorpropamide. All of these drugs occasionally produce an unusual symptom in the form of severe facial flushing after ingestion of alcohol. This can be quite marked and is socially embarrassing. It is much more common with chlorpropamide than the other drugs mentioned. In recent years there have been disturbing reports that the sulphonylureas and the diguanides (discussed below) may increase the risk of death from cardiovascular disease in 'mature onset' diabetics. As yet this has not been proven but the reports have led to reduction of the use of these

drugs in the United States. At present, however, they are still widely used in the United Kingdom.

Diguanides

There are two drugs in this group you need to know about — phenformin and metformin. Phenformin was widely used in the past but has recently fallen into disfavour because a few patients on high doses developed severe lactic acidosis — a condition which is often fatal. New patients tend to be started on metformin. These drugs do not stimulate release of insulin by the pancreas but seem to act by increasing the entry of glucose into the body cells. Hypoglycaemia is not a risk of these drugs when they are used alone but may develop if they are being used in combination with sulphonylurea agents or insulin. The diguanides do not stimulate appetite. In fact, they have anorectic effect and this makes them useful for the treatment of obese diabetics not controlled by diet alone. Occasionally when carbohydrate restriction and a sulphonylurea drug have proved unsuccessful in the treatment of diabetes, the addition of a diguanide will lower the blood sugar and obviate the need for use of insulin. Side effects are common with these drugs, nausea and diarrhoea being particularly troublesome, leading to discontinuation of treatment in a proportion of cases. As with the sulphonylureas, use of these drugs in patients with known vascular disease may constitute a hazard although this is not yet proven.

Hyperglycaemic agents

Glucagon. This is produced by the alpha cells of the pancreas and it raises blood glucose by increasing its release from the liver. It is given by subcutaneous injection to treat hypoglycaemia when it is impossible to give glucose intravenously and the patient cannot swallow glucose because he is confused or in coma. Nausea is a common side effect of this drug.

TREATMENT OF DISEASES OF THE THYROID GLAND

Iodine and thyroid hormones

The thyroid gland normally concentrates iodine from the blood and uses it in the manufacture of thyroid hormone (thyroxine).

Iodine is thus necessary for the manufacture of thyroxine. If iodine is not present in large enough amounts in the thyroid gland (because of iodine deficiency in the diet or because of the action of a drug such as potassium perchlorate which prevents the thyroid concentrating iodine from the blood stream) thyroxine will not be made.

Thyroxine is necessary for health. This hormone stimulates the metabolism of the body. In its absence or if it is present in low amounts (e.g. in the condition of thyroid underactivity, hypothyroidism) patients become listless, apathetic and dull. The skin becomes rough and dry, the hair becomes coarse and the voice croaking. The features are swollen and puffy (myxoedema) giving rise to the typical facies of a patient with *hypothyroidism*. These patients often complain that they never feel warm and they experience cold weather much more keenly than normal persons. They may develop constipation because of sluggishness of the bowel and may become slightly deaf. When thyroxine is given to patients with hypothyroidism the change in appearance which the hormone induces may be dramatic.

If thyroid hormone is present in excess as happens in *hyperthyroidism* where the thyroid gland manufactures too much thyroxine, patients complain of nervousness, irritability, breathlessness, palpitations, increased perspiration, increased appetite, loss of weight and a sense of discomfort in a warm room. These symptoms are all related to the increase in body metabolism which thyroxine induces.

A very curious and interesting fact about iodine is that in *small* amounts it is needed for the production of thyroxine but that in *large* amounts it blocks thyroxine synthesis. This knowledge was used to treat patients with hyperthyroidism before the advent of the antithyroid drugs (members of the thiourea family and potassium perchlorate). Nowadays iodine should be used only in the preoperative management of patients with hyperthyroidism who are to have a partial thyroidectomy. The action of iodine here is to render the overactive thyroid gland less vascular thus making the surgeon's task easier.

Iodine is traditionally given as Lugol's Iodine which is an aqueous solution of iodine (5 per cent) and potassium iodide (10 per cent). The dose is 0.3 ml thrice daily. Alternatively tablets of potassium iodide can be used, the dose being 60 mg thrice daily.

Occasionally patients develop reactions to iodine manifested by excess tear formation and watery nasal discharge.

Drugs used in the treatment of diseases of the thyroid gland

The commonest disorders of the thyroid gland which require drug treatment are hyperthyroidism and hypothyroidism.

Drug treatment of hyperthyroidism

The drugs most commonly used in the treatment of hyperthyroidism are members of the thiourea family. This group includes carbimazole and propylthiouracil. All of these drugs have similar actions and the one most often employed nowadays is carbimazole. This substance blocks the manufacture of thyroxine in the normal or the overactive thyroid gland. It does this by preventing iodine, the element necessary for thyroxine synthesis, from linking on to tyrosine. Blockage of this step leads to a decrease in the concentration of thyroxine in the blood. A typical dose is 15 mg three times a day for about 6 to 8 weeks when the patient usually comes under control. Thereafter the drug is given for a period of one to one and a half years in a maintenance dose of about 5 mg thrice daily. Unless the disease is mild the relapse rate of hyperthyroidism is high when carbimazole is withdrawn. If relapse does occur, the disease is then treated by radioiodine or by surgery.

The side effects of carbimazole are nausea, vomiting and skin rashes. In a few patients agranulocytosis occurs. All patients on carbimazole treatment should be instructed to stop their tablets if they develop a sore throat.

Another agent which may be used to control hyperthyroidism in patients who experience side effects with carbimazole is potassium perchlorate. This drug, like carbimazole, interferes with the manufacture of thyroxine from iodine in the thyroid gland. It does this in a different manner, by preventing the thyroid gland from concentrating iodine from the blood stream. The level of thyroxine in the blood therefore falls. Patients receiving potassium perchlorate should not be given iodine-containing medicines which could raise the concentration of iodine in the blood stream and so force iodine into the thyroid gland thus reversing the effect of potassium perchlorate. The drug is usually given in a dose of 200 mg four times a day. Agranulocytosis is a side effect of potassium perchlorate.

Beta blocking drugs in the treatment of thyrotoxicosis

Propranolol has become widely used in the treatment of thyro- toxic patients. There is an increase in adrenergic activity in this condition which is partly responsible for some of the features such as agitation, tachycardia and tremor. Beta adrenergic block- ing drugs greatly reduce these effects and provide considerable symptomatic relief. They probably have very little effect on the function of the thyroid gland itself and therefore are no substi- tute for curative therapy such as surgery ^{131}I or antithyroid drugs. Beta blockers are always used in addition to these mea- sures. The main indications for their use in thyrotoxicosis are cardiac arrhythmias such as supraventricular tachycardia and atrial fibrillation, thyroid crisis and sometimes before thyroid surgery.

Operative treatment for hyperthyroidism

This is employed if the hyperthyroid thyroid is very large or if a young patient has relapsed after treatment with drugs. Before partial thyroidectomy (the removal of about seven-eighths of thyroid) the patient should be given potassium iodide in place of carbimazole treatment for two weeks. The dose of potassium iodide is usually 60 mg three times a day. It reduces the vascular- ity of the thyroid gland and thus renders the operation technically less difficult for the surgeon. Lugol's iodine may also be used for this purpose.

Radioiodine treatment for hyperthyroidism

Sodium iodide (^{131}I) solution is used for the treatment of hyper- thyroidism mainly in patients over the age of 40 years. This substance can be administered only in specialised centres with facilities for the handling of radioactive materials. The thyroid gland cannot distinguish between [131]I (radioiodine) and [127]I (stable or non-radioactive iodine) because these substances are chemically identical. From the physical standpoint, however, each has very different properties: [131]I emits energy in the form of radiation, ^{127}I does not do this. When a patient is given a dose of ^{131}I, the thyroid concentrates the radioiodine. The energy which ^{131}I releases destroys part of the gland and brings the hyperthyroidism under control over a period of 6 to 10 weeks. Many patients treated with ^{131}I ultimately become hypothyroid. The dose of ^{131}I ranges from 7.5 to 15 mci. Doses of the order of 100 mci are sometimes given to patients with thyroid cancer in the hope that the malignant tissue will concentrate ^{131}I and be destroyed by it.

No especial precautions are needed for patients who have received less than 20 mc ^{131}I. It is a wise policy to treat hyperthyroidism with ^{131}I on an outpatient basis rather than have several patients in the same ward at the same time with consequent risk of high levels of radiation.

Patients who receive doses of the order of 100 mc for the treatment of thyroid cancer should be nursed in a side room. The nurse should wear a special lead-lined apron when she is in the room to protect her against the high level of radiation. All urine passed by the patient during the first 10 days after treatment should be stored in a special lead-lined repository until the radioactivity has decayed to safe levels (in practice 3 months are usually sufficient for radioiodine to decay to acceptable levels of radioactivity) before being disposed of.

Nursing observations on patients receiving carbimazole or potassium perchlorate

1. If a patient is receiving treatment with either of these drugs and complains of a sore throat, the matter should be reported to sister and further doses of this drug withheld pending fuller investigation (e.g. a polymorphonuclear leucocyte count).

2. If the patient is being treated as a hospital inpatient, the temperature should be taken twice daily at the start of treatment. In this way the development of an elevation of temperature in a patient with agranulocytosis may be observed early at the onset of infection.

3. The pulse rate should be recorded twice daily. You will often see a fall in the pulse rate after treatment with carbimazole or potassium perchlorate has been given for two to three weeks. Pulse rates of 120 per minute are common in patients with untreated hyperthyroidism.

4. There are a number of other observations you will be able to make for your own interest in your patient who is being treated for hyperthyroidism. These patients are often flushed and anxious looking. Many have lost a great deal of weight and show obvious signs of this and some have protrusion of the eyeballs (exophthalmos). Many of these signs clear up during treatment with antithyroid drugs.

Drug treatment of hypothyroidism

Patients with hypothyroidism lack thyroid hormone. Treatment therefore consists in giving replacement therapy with thyroxine sodium. A small dose is given (usually 0.05 mg once daily) and this is slowly increased to a maintenance dose of about 0.1 mg twice or three times daily. This can be given as a single dose in the morning. The hormone is thereafter taken indefinitely. Caution must be exercised in treating patients with angina who have hypothyroidism. There is a risk of precipitating a myocardial infarction if the dose of thyroxine sodium is increased too quickly.

If your hypothyroid patient who is being treated with thyroxine complains of tightness in the chest or complains of feeling otherwise unwell, you should report this to sister. It may be that he is being given too much thyroxine and that a reduction in dosage is called for. Patients have occasionally died following a myocardial infarction sustained while being treated with thyroxine for hypothyroidism.

DRUG TREATMENT OF DISEASES OF THE ADRENAL GLAND

Addison's disease

This condition is due to a failure of the adrenal cortex to secrete hydrocortisone. Treatment consists in giving replacement doses of oral hydrocortisone usually in doses in the range 25 to 50 mg per day. This is usually given as a divided dose, e.g. 25 mg in the morning and 12.5 mg at night. This mimicks the normal variation in cortisol levels throughout the day. Hydrocortisone is discussed in detail on p. 178. Sometimes it is necessary to give patients with Addison's disease another additional substance (such as fludrocortisone) which causes the kidneys to retain sodium. This is because the adrenal cortex normally also secretes aldosterone, a powerful sodium-retaining hormone. In Addison's disease there is failure to secrete this hormone. In many patients, however, fludrocortisone is not required because cortisone itself has some sodium-retaining properties.

DRUG TREATMENT OF DISEASES OF THE PITUITARY GLAND

The pituitary gland consists of an anterior and a posterior part. Diseases can affect one or other of both these parts.

Diseases of the anterior pituitary gland

This part of the pituitary gland secretes, among other things, thyroid stimulating hormone, adrenocortical stimulating hormone, and the hormones which stimulate the production of the sex hormones. The drug treatment of patients with hypopituitarism due to conditions affecting the anterior pituitary consists therefore of replacing thyroid hormone (p. 229), the adrenal hormone (hydrocortisone) (p. 178) and, in men, the male sex hormone (testosterone). Testosterone is discussed later. Children with dwarfism due to deficiency of growth hormone sometimes benefit from treatment with preparations of this hormone from humans. To date such preparations are not available in amounts large enough for routine use.

Diseases of the posterior pituitary gland

Patients with disorders of the posterior pituitary gland are said to be suffering from diabetes insipidus. This condition is characterised by extreme thirst and the passage of large quantities of urine. Patients with diabetes insipidus may pass more than 10 litres of urine per day. The treatment is to replace the antidiuretic hormone which is normally secreted by the posterior part of the pituitary. In health this hormone is responsible for the reabsorption in the distal kidney tubule of water which has been filtered at the glomerulus. Its absence therefore causes the passage of large quantities of dilute urine. Antidiuretic hormone has been given the name vasopressin and this drug used to be given by subcutaneous injection in the form of pitressin tannate in oil. This is no longer used for the treatment of diabetes insipidus. Most patients use lypressin or desmopressin which are administered nasally and act following absorption into the blood stream from the mucous membrane of the nasopharynx. Both drugs are synthetic forms of antidiuretic hormone but desmopressin, the newer agent, is broken down more slowly in the body and thus has a longer duration of action. It can be administered nasally once or twice a day as against lipressin which must be taken 4 to 6 hourly. It is therefore preferred in most instances. A parenteral form of desmopressin is also available which can be injected subcutaneously every 24 to 48 hours. No natural or synthetic form of antidiuretic hormone can be administered orally as it will be quickly broken down in the stomach. A fluid balance chart should be kept for the patient who is starting treatment with any form of antidiuretic hormone.

Sometimes chlorpropamide (p. 223) and carbamazepine (p. 147) are successful treatment in mild cases of diabetes insipidus. The exact means by which these drugs reduce urine output is unknown but they probably make the distal renal tubule more sensitive to the effects of what small amounts of antidiuretic hormone are still being secreted.

Oxytocin (Syntocinon)

Oxytocin is the other important hormone produced by the posterior pituitary gland. Its natural function is to stimulate expulsion of milk from the breast of suckling mothers but it also stimulates uterine contraction and this is its main therapeutic use. A synthetic form of the hormone (syntocinon) is available and this is widely used in the induction of labour. It is also valuable for the stimulation of uterine contraction in postpartum haemorrhage. Synthetic oxytocin is usually given by continuous intravenous infusion in variable doses depending on the situation. High doses can lead to violent uterine contractions and rupture. If large amounts of electrolyte free fluid are given at the same time as syntocinon then excessive retention of water may result. This condition is known as water intoxication and can lead to confusion or even coma.

Nursing observations to be made in patients receiving an intravenous infusion of oxytocin

1. Observe the uterus carefully for forcible contractions. If uterine contractions are too forcible (you will learn about this

from experience) the infusion may have to be discontinued. As soon as labour is established with regular strong contractions the administration of oxytocin is stopped.

2. The foetal heart rate should be counted regularly. If signs of foetal distress appear (a heart rate greater than 160 or less than 120 beats per minute or an irregularity of the heart rhythm) it may be necessary to stop the infusion.

Bromocriptine

This is a new drug which has been introduced for the treatment of certain endocrine diseases. It is still being evaluated but its actions are complex and may prove to be useful in the treatment of a variety of endocrine diseases. Originally, bromocriptine was introduced for the suppression of lactation as it inhibits the secretion of prolactin by the pituitary gland. It is therefore of use in suppressing lactation following pregnancy and in some other disorders when lactation occurs outside pregnancy and is sometimes associated with amenorrhoea. Bromocriptine also inhibits the secretion of growth hormone and it may be useful in the medical treatment of patients suffering from the rare condition known as acromegaly. This condition results from excessive secretion of growth hormone by a tumour of the pituitary gland. More recently, bromocriptine has also been found useful in the treatment of Parkinson's disease. It must be stressed that the drug is currently used only by specialists and side effects, in particular nausea and vomiting, seem to be quite common.

FEMALE SEX HORMONES

A full discussion of the female sex hormones is outside the scope of this book. There are two female sex hormones, oestrogen and progesterone, which are produced by the ovaries. Oestrogen is secreted by the Graafian follicle in the ovary and progesterone by the corpus luteum.

Oestrogen

The term oestrogen embraces a number of naturally occurring and synthetic hormones with many actions. These are as follows:

1. Proliferation of the endometrium of the uterus in the first 14 days of the menstrual cycle
2. Development in the female of the secondary sexual characteristics at puberty
3. Maintance of the normal structure of the female reproductive tract
4. Inhibition of lactation and ovulation (in large doses).

Uses of oestrogen

1. Menopausal symptoms such as flushing and anxiety which are due to acute deprivation of oestrogen at the menopause are relieved by the administation of oestrogen
2. Dysmenorrhoea is more common when ovulation has occurred. Oestrogen suppresses ovulation and use of an oestrogen containing contraceptive pill will effectively relieve the pain of dysmenorrhoea
3. Carcinoma of the prostate and carcinoma of the breast sometimes regress for a short time if oestrogen is administered.
4. Lactation is inhibited by large doses of oestrogen. Mothers who do not want to breast feed their infants can be given oestrogens to suppress lactation. Other forms of treatment for suppression of lactation are available. One of the most modern forms of therapy is with a new drug called Bromocriptine (see section on bromocriptine therapy). Diuretics are sometimes prescribed in this situation. These drugs do not prevent lactation but effectively relieve the symptoms associated with painful engorgements of the breast.

Substances with oestrogenic activity

Stilboestrol is a synthetic substance with oestrogenic activity. It is given orally, the dose depending on the condition being treated and varying from 0.1 to 25 mg daily. It causes nausea and vomiting in a very high proportion of women.

Ethinyloestradiol is the most potent oestrogenic substance known. It is given orally and is some 25 times more active than stilboestrol.

Oestradiol occurs naturally in the body but must be given to patients parenterally. It is used if the other preparations cause vomiting.

Progestogens

These hormones have the following actions:

1. They prepare the endometrium of the uterus for implantation of the fertilised ovum in the second 14 days of the menstrual cycle
2. They maintain the health of the placenta in early pregnancy and the health of the uterine lining throughout pregnancy
3. Progesterone acting in conjunction with oestrogen can either stimulate or inhibit the secretion of the pituitary gonadotrophic hormones depending on the doses used. These two substances can thus be used together to inhibit ovulation. This is the mechanism of action of the oral contraceptives.

Uses of progesterone

1. Metropathia haemorrhagica is a disease characterised by heavy uterine bleeding. This condition is associated with failure of ovulation and is caused by excessive and prolonged stimulation of the endometrium by oestrogen. Progesterone is administered to patients with this disease some 12 days after the end of a spell of abnormal endometrial bleeding and will induce more normal menstruation a few days later
2. The value of progesterone in the teatment of habitual obortion is not yet certain. Treatment is sometimes given to patients who have had recurrent abortion in the hope that the exogenously administered progesterone will help maintain the developing placenta
3. When oestrogen and progesterone are given together in suitable doses at the correct time, they inhibit the secretion of the pituitary gonadotrophic hormones and thus inhibit ovulation. These drugs therefore exert a contraceptive effect.

Substances with progestational activity

Norethisterone is a valuable progestational agent which is given by mouth. A typical dose is 5 mg thrice daily. This drug is a derivative of the male sex hormone testosterone.

Hydroxyprogesterone is a progesterone derivative used in the treatment of habitual abortion. Its value is uncertain.

Drugs used for the control of conception

At present oral contraceptives are only available for women although preparations for men are being evaluated. There are four types of oral contraceptive.

1. Combined preparations.

These are by far the most widely used and contain a progestogen and an oestrogen. The exact type and proportion used varies from one product to another, so one preparation may suit one woman better than another. The tablets are commenced on the fifth day after the start of menstruation and are taken for 21 days. After a break of 7 days the course is repeated. Menstruation usually starts 2 to 5 days after stopping the tablets. It is usually advised that another method of contraception should be used during the first month as suppression of ovulation is not guaranteed. Most women notice a reduction in blood loss while on the pill and it is quite common for bleeding to be absent during one or two cycles.

2. Sequential preparations

These are not used as frequently as in the past. Oestrogen is given from day 5 to 21 of the cycle and this is followed by oestrogen plus a progestogen for the next 7 days. The main advantage of this form of preparation is that some women find it easier when they have to take a pill every day. When there is a gap in treatment as with the combined preparations they sometimes have difficulty remembering to re-start on the right day. The risks of sequential preparations are the risks of any oestrogen containing drug (see below).

3. Progestogen-only pills

These act mainly by altering the character of the cervical mucous, making it difficult for spermatozoa to penetrate. They are less effective than combined preparations and are taken every day throughout the menstrual cycle. The risks associated with taking low dose progestogen preparations are less than oestrogen containing drugs and they may on occasion be used when an oestrogen preparation is contra-indicated (see below).

4. Depot contraceptives

This form of treatment has fairly limited use. A combination of oestrogen and progestogen or progestogen only may be given in a sustained release form by 3 monthly intramuscular injection.

Hazards of oral contraceptives

First of all, it must be said that the much publicised risks of oral contraceptives are very small when considered by the individual patient. There is a definite increase in the risk of development of deep vein thrombosis or myocardial infarction and this fact must be taken into account whenever an oral contraceptive preparation is prescribed. Thrombosis of the deep veins of the leg with resulting pulmonary embolism is more likely if the patient is immobilised for any length of time, for instance, during surgery, but these complications also develop in otherwise healthy young women. It is probably related to the dose of oestrogen in the pill and is less of a risk with low dose preparations containing $30\mu g$ of oestrogen or less.

The increased risk of stroke and myocardial infarction is a recent discovery and it is not possible to say whether low-dose preparations are safer. Certainly older women who have been on the pill for a long time are at greater risk, and cigarette smoking almost certainly increases the hazard. Other less well known hazards are an increase in the incidence of gall-bladder disease and an otherwise very rare condition — benign adenoma of the liver. It is important to point out that there is no definite increase in the risk of development of any form of malignant disease amongst women who use the contraceptive pill. Most women experience a slight rise in blood pressure when starting the pill. In a few this becomes frankly abnormal and necessitates discontinuation of therapy.

Most of the hazards enumerated above seem to be related to the oestrogen content of the pill and low-dose preparations are probably safer. It is possible that the risk of hypertension is in part related to the progestogen content. Minor side effects in patients recently started on the pill, for instance, weight gain, slight nausea and breast discomfort are quite common and usually disappear in time. On occasions, a change to a preparation containing a different balance of oestrogen and progestogen is helpful.

When considering the risks of the contraceptive pill it is also necessary to consider the benefits. The pill is certainly more effective than other forms of contraception so the risks of accidental pregnancy are lessened. Menstruation is regulated and usually painless and the incidence of benign diseases of the breast and ovary is reduced.

As many of the hazards of oral contraceptive use have been identified, it is now possible to single out those who are at greatest risk. The pill can be regarded as safe in otherwise healthy young women with normal blood pressure. In older women (over the age of 35 years) who smoke, it is reasonable to consider some other form of contraception but the pill is certainly not completely contraindicated. Women over the age of 40 who have been on the pill for a long time and smoke should certainly be advised to use some other form of contraception. Clearly, there is a need for a careful, individual assessment of the possible risks in each case before the pill is prescribed.

Contraindications to use of the contraceptive pill

1. Carcinoma of the breast or genital tract is an absolute contraindication
2. A history of thrombosis is an absolute contraindication
3. High blood pressure is an absolute contraindication
4. Patients with severe varicose veins should be advised to use other forms of contraception
5. The pill probably should not be prescribed to patients who have suffered from certain forms of jaundice but a history of uncomplicated hepatitis certainly should not prevent use.

Drugs used to increase fertility

Clomiphine

Clomiphine stimulates the secretion of pituitary gonadotrophins and is used in the treatment of infertility due to failure of ovulation. The major risk is of inducing multiple pregnancy.

Gonadotrophins

Human gonadotrophin has been administered to stimulate ovulation in cases of infertility. In some cases it has been dramatically successful but the risk of multiple birth is very high and this form of treatment is being used less frequently nowadays.

MALE SEX HORMONES

Male sex hormones, known as androgens, are substances which cause masculinisation. Their main uses are in restoring secondary sex characteristics to castrated males or to male patients with hypopituitarism who have failure of secretion of the pituitary gonadotrophins. Androgens are of value in the treatment of some cases of inoperable breast carcinoma especially in patients before the menopause and especially if bony metastases are present. As you might expect, the male sex hormones cause increases in muscle mass and in the rate of growth of the skeleton. These hormones stimulate the build-up of body protein. They are often used in the treatment of patients with osteoporosis in the hope that they may promote an increase in the protein matrix of thin bones. They are also given occasionally to patients with acute renal failure in an attempt to decrease protein breakdown and thus ease the burden of the kidneys in excreting the end products of protein metabolism.

Preparations of male sex hormones

Testosterone which is the natural hormone secreted by the testis must be given parenterally. The effect of one 25 mg injection of testosterone propionate given by intramuscular injection may last for a week. Alternatively pellets of this preparation may be implanted under the skin in a dose sufficient to last the patient 6 months or longer.

Fluoxymesterone has androgenic activity when given by mouth. A typical dose is in the range 1 to 5 mg daily. Norethandrolone is more active as an anabolic agent than as an androgenic drug. The compound does produce side virilising effects, however, such as promoting increased growth of facial hair and deepening of the voice when it is used in women. It is given orally in a dose of 10 to 30 mg per day. Nandrolone is an anabolic agent suitable for parenteral use. The effect of a 25 mg injection lasts for one to two weeks.

Tamoxifen

Tamoxifen is not really a male sex hormone. It acts as an antagonist to oestrogen, the female hormone. It is used as an alternative to androgens in the management of advanced breast cancer.

MISCELLANEOUS DRUGS

Prostaglandins

These are naturally occurring substances found throughout the body which have many different actions. They may be used either alone or in combination with oxytocin for induction of labour or therapeutic abortion. For termination of pregnancy, they may be given either directly into the uterus or intravenously. High doses are required and nausea, vomiting, diarrhoea and abdominal pain are common side effects. When the drugs are given in lower doses intravenously for the induction of labour, side effects are less common. (See also p. 170).

12

Intravenous fluid therapy

Intravenous fluids are widely prescribed for medical and surgical patients. Although they are seldom considered in the same category as drugs, parenteral fluids are extremely hazardous if used in a careless or casual fashion. Although fluids are prescribed by medical staff, nurses have complete control over their administration and it seems wise to consider in detail the types of fluids used and the special problems associated with this form of therapy. This chapter will cover the commonly used basic intravenous solutions but will not cover the specialised topics of blood transfusion and parenteral nutrition.

INDICATIONS FOR I.V. FLUID THERAPY

Intravenous fluids are indicated either for the 'replacement' of sudden fluid losses or the 'maintenance' of normal fluid balance in patients who are unable to do this by the natural oral route.

Replacement therapy

The indications for fluid replacement are usually fairly clear and the choice of fluid required will guided by the clinical problem. It is obvious that sudden haemorrhage is best treated by rapid replacement of fresh blood. If this is not available, plasma protein solution will often be used. Normal (0.9 per cent) saline is always available and this is usually the first fluid administered following haemorrhage, that is until properly matched blood is available. Patients who have lost large amounts of fluid and electrolytes, for instance as a result of severe diarrhoea, intestinal obstruction or diabetic ketoacidosis, require replacement with normal saline and the great majority will also need potassium added to the solution. Potassium supplements are often withheld until the patient's blood level is reported as low by the laboratory. This is foolish as the great majority of patients will require 60 mmol per day, and possibly much more if they start with a deficit. The body is very poor at conserving potassium and an attempt should always be made to anticipate this need. An exception to this rule is the patient with advanced renal failure for whom potassium must always be prescribed with great care.

Sometimes patients develop pure dehydration, in other words they become deficient in body water. This can occur as a result of pyrexia, renal disease, inadequate intake of water over a long period or sometimes in elderly diabetics. It is not possible to infuse large amounts of pure water intravenously as haemolysis and death will result. Instead, dehydration is corrected with 5 per cent dextrose. This contains no electrolytes and the sugar content is very quickly metabolised leaving pure water. If it seems undesirable to administer dextrose to a dehydrated patient, for instance in diabetes, half strength (0.45 per cent) saline may be given. This contains a much lower concentration of sodium than plasma, so effectively provides the patient with additional water.

When any patient requires rapid fluid replacement, it is important to decide whether the primary need is for fluid and electrolytes or fluid alone. This decision is based on a careful consideration of the history, clinical findings and blood biochemistry. You will note that the above account only mentions saline solutions, dextrose and potassium. This may seem surprising as a vast array of complex electrolyte solutions is available. The simple truth is that the great majority of clinical problems can be managed with combinations of these fluids and the use of complicated mixed solutions is unnecessary and potentially confusing.

Maintenance therapy

When normal oral intake of fluid and electrolytes is impossible, for instance after abdominal surgery or during coma, the intravenous route has to supply the maintenance needs of the body. With the exception of patients suffering from renal or cardiac failure, most patients need at least two litres of fluid per day while in hospital. They also need around 150 mmol of sodium each day. The body conserves sodium very effectively, so precise replacement is not vital. Potassium replacement must be undertaken with care and assuming that there are no excessive losses, for instance from fistulae, approximately 60 to 80 mmol is needed in 24 hours. So, in practice, a regime consisting of 1 to 1.5 litres of 5 per cent dextrose and 0.5 to 1.0 litre of 0.9 per cent saline with added potassium chloride will provide the maintenance requirements of the majority of patients.

SOLUTIONS IN COMMON USE

Saline solutions

Normal saline

0.9 per cent saline contains 154 mmol mmol of sodium and chloride ions per litre. This means that it has a slightly higher sodium content than normal plasma and it must be given with great care to patients in cardiac failure who have already a tendency to sodium retention. As noted above, normal saline is most often used to replace fluid and electrolyte losses.

Half strength saline (0.45 per cent)

This solution contains 74 mmol of sodium per litre. In other words approximately half that of normal plasma. It is not commonly used, but may be administered instead of dextrose for the treatment of dehydration.

Double strength saline (1.8 per cent)

1.8 per cent saline and even higher concentrations are available but are seldom used. Their main indication is severe life-threatening sodium depletion. You will often see patient's serum sodium levels reported as low. This usually indicates fluid retention by the body with dilution of the blood rather than true sodium deficiency. The use of highly concentrated saline in this situation is wrong. Occasionally when the serum sodium is extremely low and accompanied by drowsiness or coma, high strength saline solutions are infused slowly but this must be done with great care.

Carbohydrate solutions

Dextrose 5 per cent

This is very commonly used to provide water for patients unable to swallow. This solution is very safe and is less likely to induce cardiac failure in susceptible individuals than saline solutions. The nutrient value is low (190 calories per litre) but may result in hyperglycaemia if given to diabetics. It is not commonly appreciated that dextrose solutions are acidic and therefore tend to irritate veins which results in phlebitis.

Higher strength dextrose solutions

Dextrose solutions with strengths varying from 10 per cent to 50 per cent (380 to 1900 calories per litre) are available. The 50 per cent solution is invaluable for correcting hypoglycaemia in diabetics. It is also used to feed seriously ill patients, for example, in liver failure. Five to ten per cent solutions can be infused into arm veins but 20 to 50 per cent solutions must be given through long intravenous catheters sited in the superior or inferior venae cava. This is because of their high viscosity and tendency to produce severe phlebitis.

Fructose

You will seldom see fructose used. It is a convenient calorie source as the body cells can metabolise it without the assistance of insulin. Unfortunately when it is given in large amounts it leads to the accumulation of lactic acid in the body. This may lead to serious metabolic disturbance.

Alkaline solutions

Sodium bicarbonate

This is the most convenient solution for the correction of metabolic acidosis as it supplies the body with its natural buffer—bicarbonate. The 8.4 per cent solution is usually available and this conveniently contains 100 mmol in 100 ml. If large amounts, for instance 200 ml or more, of this solution are administered very quickly during cardiac arrest or forced alkaline diuresis, too rapid correction of the patient's metabolic upset may result and this can be dangerous. The 1.43 per cent solution is safer in most instances but as it contains only 170 mmol of sodium bicarbonate per litre the large volume that must be infused makes it impractical for the management of cardiac arrest.

Sodium lactate

Normal individuals convert lactate to bicarbonate which helps to combat acidosis. This conversion may be impaired in ill patients and it is possible for lactate to accumulate in the blood. A number of intravenous solutions contain lactate and it is important that you should always know their constituents before giving them to patients. It is difficult to see any advantage in using these fluids and in general it is best to confine use to 5 per cent dextrose and 0.9 per cent saline in appropriate combinations.

Acid solutions

Occasionally it is necessary to give an acidic solution to a patient to correct severe alkalosis. This most often results from prolonged vomiting in pyloric stenosis which leads to loss of large amounts of acid from the stomach. Saline and potassium chloride help to correct this state but an infusion of ammonium chloride is sometimes given in severe cases. Occasionally dilute hydrochloric acid has been given but this is fairly hazardous.

INTRAVENOUS POTASSIUM THERAPY

Potassium chloride is usually provided as a solution which contains 2 mmol per ml. This highly concentrated solution must *never* be injected directly as hyperkalaemia and death from cardiac arrest will almost certainly result. Instead the solution is mixed into infusion bags or bottles, usually giving a concentration of 40 mmol per litre. Some patients, for instance during treatment of severe diabetic coma, require large amounts of potassium and this may have to be given in doses greater than 20 mmol per hour. This should only be done with very careful monitoring of the serum potassium level. In routine circumstances, patients should not receive potassium in doses greater than 5 mmol per hour. It is important, therefore, that you should not 'speed up' an infusion containing potassium which is running late in order to keep it to time. When potassium chloride is added to the flexible fluid containers in the upright position, i.e. hanging from the drip stand, it may 'pool' in high concentrations at the bottom of the bag. If this solution is then infused quickly, death from hyperkalaemia may result. It is necessary to remove the bag from the stand and ensure proper mixing after addition of potassium to the fluid. Only then should the fluid be administered to the patient. Because of this problem infusion fluids are now available which already contain potassium chloride mixed in with dextrose or saline by the fluid manufacturer. These fluids are widely used and are safer so long as the nursing and medical staff know exactly what the potassium content of the fluid is. Care must be taken not to administer such fluids in error to patients who do not in fact require potassium.

CALCIUM SALTS

Calcium is given intravenously only when very rapid correction of hypocalcaemia is necessary. An example of this is severe tetany with convulsions due to calcium deficiency. Two solutions, calcium gluconate and calcium chloride are generally available. Calcium gluconate is preferred as it is much less irritating to tissues. If calcium chloride leaks from an injection site it can lead to tissue necrosis. Injections of calcium must be given slowly as cardiac arrhythmias can occur. Calcium salts must not be injected simultaneously with sodium bicarbonate, as calcium carbonate will instantly form. This will result in the patient receiving an injection of chalk!

MIXED INTRAVENOUS SOLUTIONS

A large number of mixed solutions are available. In general they offer no advantage over plain dextrose or saline solutions.

Pre-mixed potassium solutions

These have already been discussed in the section on potassium therapy.

Ringer's solution

This is a fairly popular fluid which in essence is saline, with the addition of a small amount of potassium and calcium. It has no possible advantage over normal saline, as the amount of potassium is so small that it does not come anywhere near meeting the patient's requirement. The reasons for its popularity remain a mystery.

Ringer lactate

This is Ringer's solution with the addition of lactate. This solution has the limitations of plain Ringer's solution with the additional problem that lactate administration to an ill patient may be hazardous (see section on alkaline solutions). For these reasons the solution is not recommended.

Dextrose saline mixtures

A number of solutions in varying concentrations are available. The solution containing 0.18 per cent saline and 4 per cent dextrose is the most useful as it has approximately the same osmolarity as plasma with only a low sodium content. Other mixtures, particularly that containing 0.9 per cent saline and 5 per cent dextrose, are not recommended as they are very concentrated solutions and have no possible advantage.

'Balanced' electrolyte solutions

You will occasionally see fluids used which have complex constituents and claim to contain balanced quantities of electrolytes. There is no such thing as a 'balanced' solution. What the patient receives should be determined by what the patient requires and these needs can always met be a combination of water (5 per cent dextrose), electrolyte (0.9 per cent saline) and potassium chloride in carefully calculated amounts. The appropriate quantities must be determined by proper clinical and biochemical assessment. When you are asked to administer a mixed solution to a patient, please ensure that both you and the medical staff know what the fluid contains.

HAZARDS OF INTRAVENOUS FLUID THERAPY

The risks of parenteral fluid therapy are often forgotten. It is generally assumed that intravenous solutions are completely safe and therefore can be used with impunity. In fact, they result in side effects as often as many drugs and should therefore be used with equal care. There is no excuse for careless procedure either during the 'setting up' of an infusion or during its supervision. The following section outlines the general hazards of intravenous fluid therapy. It does not lay down rules about correct administration techniques. This information must be obtained from your nursing procedures manual. The adverse effects described are those of the fluids themselves. Clearly if a drug is added to an infusion and delivered intravenously, then the additional hazards of the drug itself must also be considered.

Thrombophlebitis

It is widely assumed that inflammation and thrombosis of a vein used for an infusion indicates infection. This is not so. Phlebitis usually develops as a result of irritation of the endothelium (inner lining of the vein). This can either be physical damage by the intravenous cannula or chemical irritation by the infusion fluid or its contents. In this latter respect, dextrose solutions are the main culprits because of their acidity. The risk of phlebitis increases the longer the cannula is left in position and this painful complication will eventually occur in all cases if the infusion site is not changed. Although bacteria themselves do not usually cause phlebitis the inflamed vein and blood clot provide an ideal breeding site and secondary infection can result. This can lead to severe suppurative phlebitis, which may result in spread of organisms into the blood stream (septicaemia). When phlebitis occurs, the infusion should be discontinued. Antibiotics do not have to be given routinely for this complication. Thrombosis of the veins of the arm only rarely results in dissemination of blood clot into the lungs (pulmonary embolism), but this serious complication is a real risk if an intravenous infusion is positioned in the veins of the foot or lower legs. These sites should never be used.

Infection

If infection complicates the use of intravenous fluids, it is potentially serious, as the organisms have a direct access to the circulation. Many potential sources of infection arise during the manufacture and use of intravenous fluids.

Contamination of the Cannula

Normal skin bacteria are frequent contaminants of intravenous catheters and adequate sterilisation of skin of operator and patient prior to venepuncture is essential. The setting up of an intravenous infusion must always be treated as a sterile procedure. Proprietary antiseptic solutions are usually effective if used in the right concentrations. Shaving of the skin is unnecessary and may increase the risk of contamination by alteration of the normal skin flora. Infection seems to be commoner when infusion is sited in the lower limbs and is a much more frequent problem when an infusion is left in the same site for a long time. For this reason catheters positioned in the superior or inferior vena cava are a particular risk, as they may be left in position for weeks or months. Bacterial or fungal infections of such infusions have resulted in the death of a number of patients. If you are asked to assist in the insertion of a central venous catheter, you must do your utmost to ensure the sterility of the procedure

Thrombophlebitis

Infection may complicate phlebitis. This is discussed fully in the preceding section (p. 247).

Contamination of infusion fluid or administration set

Bacterial contamination has occasionally occurred during manufacture of intravenous fluids and has resulted in disastrous outbreaks of septicaemia. Such events are happily very rare as commercial sterilisation techniques are strictly supervised. The appearance of the fluid is no guide to the presence of infection as it will be perfectly clear unless heavy contamination is present. It is obvious however that a fluid which is even slightly cloudy should *never* be administered to a patient. Contamination of infusion fluids is much more likely as a result of cracks or punctures of fluid containers and may also result from any procedure which involves injection of drugs into the bottle or administration set. Infection is more likely if the administration set is left unchanged for long periods. For these reasons, it is important that you should follow these rules:

a. Inspect any fluid very carefully
b. Inspect the container for cracks or puncture
c. Reduce injections into the container or administration set to an absolute minimum and ensure that a proper sterile technique is employed. Better still, have the drug added under sterile conditions by the pharmacy staff
d. Ensure that the administration set is changed every 24 hours. These precautions have been shown to reduce the risk of this serious and potentially fatal complication of intravenous fluid theraphy.

Fluid overload

When intravenous fluids are infused into healthy individuals in excessive amounts the increase in venous return to the heart stimulates cardiac output and renal bloodflow. The solute content of the fluid may have an osmotic effect on the renal tubules and the excessive load of fluid and electolytes will depress secretion of antidiuretic hormone by the pituitary gland and aldosterone by the kidney (these hormones are responsible for retention of water and salt by the body). These actions result in very high urine flow rates which ensure that enough water and electrolyte are excreted through the kidneys to prevent overload. Most patients, however, have some abnormality of at least one of the mechanisms described above. The elderly and those suffering from diseases of the heart and kidneys are particularly at risk and fluid overload will result, causing oedema of the peripheries and lungs, or hypertension. Such patients should be treated with great care as pulmonary oedema when it occurs may be fatal, despite diuretic therapy. Intravenous fluids are best avoided in these circumstances, unless they are essential to the welfare of the patient. Saline solutions are a particular risk as sodium handling by the body is often defective.

You should carefully monitor the pulse and blood pressure of all patients receiving intravenous fluids. A careful record of fluid intake and output and weight is essential. You should regularly examine the legs and sacral areas for signs of oedema and report this if present. Under no circumstances should an infusion be run through extra quickly in order to make up time.

Air embolism

When a large amount of air enters a vein it is carried to the heart and may cause death by blocking the outlet of the right side of the heart. This is known as acute cor pulmonale. The amount of air required to do this is in fact large—around 200 ml—and it has to be injected into the vein quickly. It is virtually impossible for such a large amount of air to be introduced through a modern flexible infusion set sited in the arm, as no airway is used and the fluid is not driven under pressure. If, however, the cannula is being sited in the internal jugular or subclavian veins, the danger is a real one. This is because there may be negative pressure in these vessels if the patient is shocked and is placed in an upright or semi-upright position. When the hollow cannula is inserted into the vessel the air may be sucked in surprising quickly with fatal results. The greatest risk is during insertion, or subsequently if the administration set becomes dislodged from the hub of the cannula by accident. For this reason it is essential that central venous cannulae are inserted with the patient tilted in a head-down position. It is most important that the administration set is well secured and you must check regularly to see that it is firmly connected to the cannula.

The above section describes in some detail the major complications of intravenous fluid therapy. Many of these complications are potentially fatal and this means that parenteral fluids are amongst the most dangerous drugs administered to patients in hospitals. While adverse reactions to some drugs are unavoidable and are the price we pay for effective therapy, the hazards of intravenous fluids can be averted if this form of therapy is restricted to those who really need it and the administration of fluids is treated with the respect and care it deserves.

13

Adverse drug reactions and drug interactions

It is important to understand that all effective drugs are potential poisons. With most it is mainly a question of dosage. Adverse or unwanted effects in a proportion of patients is the price we pay for efficacious therapy. In fact, modern drugs are remarkably safe and very few patients become seriously ill or die directly as a result of drugs used for therapeutic purposes. Such serious adverse reactions that do occur nearly always involve patients who are already ill and are usually being treated for conditions which themselves are potentially fatal. In determining whether unwanted effects do occur the manner in which the drug is used and the particular susceptibility of the individual patient are often more important than the inherent toxicity of the drug itself. More thought will be given to this later.

As a general rule the severity of adverse effects from an individual drug will vary according to the condition it is being used to treat. For instance, the side effects of cytotoxic drug therapy (usually bone marrow depression) are common and serious but are acceptable given that the patients are suffering from an ultimately fatal condition and such therapy is likely to prolong life and relieve distressing symptoms. Such serious adverse affects would be completely unacceptable with a drug which is likely to be widely used for treatment of a trivial condition, for instance an antibacterial agent used for upper respiratory infections. This must be very safe over a wide range of dosages.

Much is known about the adverse effects produced by drugs which have been in use for many years. The accumulated experience of generations of doctors is contained in the standard textbooks on medicine and therapeutics. In some cases it has taken a long time to learn about the toxicity of these drugs and how best to avoid it. Society demands much greater safety from new drugs and special methods have therefore been devised to identify toxicity at an early stage. Regulations governing the release of new drugs are very strict indeed and drug companies have to produce a great deal of information on the safety and efficacy of their products before a licence will be issued. Despite these precautions serious side effects can develop some years after introduction of a new drug and lead to its withdrawal. The eye damage produced by practolol is an example of this (see Ch. 3, p. 58). The reason for this is that relatively uncommon and unexpected toxicity may not be identified until many thousands of patients have taken the drug for long periods. For this reason schemes are now being introduced to monitor large numbers of recipients of new drugs in the community. The hope is that this will speed the identification of serious toxicity from drugs in the future. It is not yet clear whether this hope will be realised.

The common side effects of most drugs have been covered in the relevant sections of this book. It is necessary, however, to discuss in more detail the different ways in which drugs can produce adverse effects and how they can be prevented.

TYPES OF ADVERSE REACTION

Extension of therapeutic effect

The unwanted effects of many drugs are in reality an extension or exaggeration of their normal action. Examples are hypoglycaemia due to insulin, asthma due to beta-adrenergic blocking drugs, coma due to morphine or other potent sedatives, and haemorrhage due to anticoagulants. In some cases an overdose of the drug is the reason and in others it has been a failure to appreciate that the patient's condition has rendered him unduly susceptible to the effects of the drug. Patients with hepatic failure, for instance, are remarkably sensitive to morphine, even in small doses. It is wrong to call these toxic effects, as the drug itself is seldom to blame. The importance of this group of unwanted effects is that they are preventable. Some thought given to the question of correct dosage and the particular weaknesses of the individual patient will be rewarded by fewer accidents.

Drug idiosyncrasy

Occasionally an apparently otherwise normal individual will exhibit a remarkably exaggerated response to a small dose of a drug. Examples are, serious cardiac arrhythmias produced by quinidine or a more recent example, severe hypotension produced by small doses of the antihypertensive drug, prazosin. Some drugs seem more likely than others to produce idiosyncrasy and for the two examples given it has become practice to administer small test doses of the drug prior to commencing therapy. The term idiosyncrasy used to be used more often than it is today. Research into drug action and the ways by which the body handles drugs has revealed that many of the so-called hypersensitivity reactions are due simply to retention of the drug in the body, for instance digoxin accumulation due to kidney failure. Many old people are said to be 'sensitive' to digoxin. In many cases this toxicity is mainly due to excessive amounts of digoxin in the body. It is not adequately appreciated that the kidneys of an elderly individual do not work as well as those of a 20-year-old and the dose of digoxin must be reduced (see p. 36).

Allergic reactions to drugs

A large number of compounds are capable of producing allergic responses in a proportion of patients receiving them. Some are renowned for this tendency, particularly the penicillin group. The type of reaction may vary from acute anaphylaxis causing shock, laryngeal oedema and sometimes death following an injection of benzylpenicillin, to the more familiar and less serious problem of the rash that develops in around 8 per cent patients who are prescribed ampicillin. In these reactions the drug molecules are thought to combine with proteins in the blood stream to form 'haptens' which then stimulate an antibody response and lead to release of histamine and other chemicals which produce vasodilatation. If the individual is 're-challenged' with the same drug at a later date the reaction may be very much more severe as the patient's immune system has already been sensitised to the drug. With other drugs the body's allergic responses may be delayed and the clinical features quite different. Sulphonamides occasionally result in a generalised upset characterised by fever and joint pains. It is not so easily recognised as the characteristic penicillin rash and may be mistaken for a systemic illness. Less well understood are the cases of ocular and cutaneous damage developing in recipients of the beta-blocking drug practolol, and the occasional individual who develops a condition very like systemic lupus erythematosis after exposure to hydrallazine (p. 73) or procainamide (p. 51). It is certain that some disturbance of the body's immune system is responsible for these reactions but the mechanisms are not well understood.

DRUG INTERACTIONS

Much attention has been directed towards the ways in which one drug can alter the patient's response to another being prescribed at the same time. Many books have been written about the subject and complicated charts devised warning of the hazards of drug A and drug B taken together. Of course the golden rule when prescribing is to use as few drugs as possible whatever the indication for treatment, but in some cases simultaneous prescription of three or four drugs is unavoidable and in the majority of cases no serious problems develop. There are many theoretical sites at which drug interactions could occur but it is only fair to point out that in only a few instances are these of any great clinical significance. The more important drug interactions are listed below. Interactions between drugs can occur at any stage of passage through the body:

1. Sites outside the body
2. At the site of absorption
3. At the sites of transport or storage
4. At the site of action
5. At sites where drugs are metabolised

Interactions at sites outside the body

Drug interactions outside the body occur chiefly with substances in solution. A few examples of this follow.

Protamine zinc insulin and soluble insulin

If both of these substances are drawn up into the same syringe some of the excess protamine in the protamine zinc insulin will react with the soluble insulin and convert it into a longer-acting form of insulin. The result is that your patient's diabetic control may be poor because he will have less shorter-acting soluble insulin than he should and more longer-acting insulin than he should. This interaction can be potentially dangerous because hypoglycaemia may occur during the night when your patient is asleep.

Thiopentone and suxamethonium

Both drugs are widely used in anaesthetic practice, the first to establish anaesthesia rapidly, the second as a muscle relaxant. They must not be drawn up in the same syringe because they react chemically with each other.

Interactions at the site of absorption

Drugs which affect the motility of the alimentary tract may increase or decrease absorption of other drugs. For example, agents such as atropine, propantheline (p. 18) benzhexol (p. 150) and morphine (p. 161) decrease the movements of the bowel, delay emptying of the stomach and may thus reduce the rate and extent of absorption of other drugs.

Tetracycline and metallic ions

Tetracyclines combine very readily with metal ions such as calcium, magnesium and iron. The resulting compound is insoluble and is not absorbed. Thus the patient given even a small dose of oral ferrous sulphate for anaemia and oral tetracycline for a co-existing infection may fail to show a response to either treatment. As most proprietary antacid preparations contain magnesium or aluminium, and tetracyclines are widely prescribed this is a potentially common interaction.

Oral anticoagulants and broad spectrum antibacterial agents

Vitamin K which antagonises the action of oral anticoagulants is sythesised to some extent by bacteria in the colon. When a patient is started on anticoagulants, therapy is given until a balance is achieved between his natural resistance (produced in part by the synthesis of vitamin K by the bacteria in the gut) to these agents and his sensitivity. If antibacterial drugs are given later, they kill the bacterial flora and consequently produce a fall in the amount of vitamin K being produced. The patient's resistance to his anticoagulants decreases sharply and he is then liable to bleed.

At sites of transport or storage

A few drugs interact directly in the plasma. For example protamine neutralises heparin and this is an interaction which is of benefit to the patient (p. 198). More common and clinically important are interactions concerned with the transport of drugs on plasma albumen. (p. 2).

Warfarin and aspirin, phenylbutazone and indomethacin

There are a number of sites on albumen that may carry drugs. Some agents are carried on these sites in preference to others. For example aspirin is carried in preference to warfarin and so is phenylbutazone, oxyphenbutazone and indomethacin. If a patient is being treated with warfarin (or for that matter phenindione) and is subsequently given aspirin, there will be a deterioration of his anticoagulant control and a likelihood of severe and perhaps fatal haemorrhage. This is because the aspirin is preferentially taken up by the albumen and displaces the warfarin that was previously bound there. Unbound warfarin is active, bound drug is not (p. 2). Therefore when there is an increase in the amount of warfarin in the plasma that is unbound, the patient is more likely to bleed.

Similar considerations hold for the effect of phenylbutazone and its derivative oxyphenbutazone and indomethacin. Whenever you have a patient on anticoagulants, therefore, you must explain to him how important it is that he takes no medicines other than those prescribed by the doctor. Now many patients do not think of aspirin as a 'drug' because familiarity with this agent over many years has led them to the belief that it is a safe household remedy (which in the majority of cases admittedly it is). Thus aspirin should be one of the drugs that you should specify quite precisely as being dangerous because it may increase the bleeding tendency.

Some patients have died because of the interaction of warfarin and the drugs mentioned above. Another dangerous interaction of a different sort involving anticoagulants is discussed later (p. 259).

Interactions at the site of action

Many drugs act on a specific part of the body (for example, a nerve ending) and are selectively concentrated where they are to act. The site at which the drug is taken up is usually called the receptor site and just as there is preferential uptake by plasma albumen of one drug as opposed to another so the receptor site may display a variable affinity for different drugs. If the site is occupied by one drug for which it has a high affinity, it will be unable to take up a second drug for which it has a lower affinity (p. 3).

Some drugs combine with the receptor site and stimulate it to act. For example, isoprenaline combines with receptor sites in the heart and causes tachycardia and increased force of contraction of the heart muscle leading to an increase in blood pressure. Other drugs combine with the receptor site and merely prevent other agents becoming attached without in any way stimulating the site to act. Thus the site has become blocked. For example, propranolol (p. 54) combines with receptor sites in the heart and prevents isoprenaline from becoming attached to the same sites. If isoprenaline is given to a patient who has received propranolol previously, the rise expected in pulse rate and blood pressure does not occur.

Morphine and naloxone

Naloxone is taken up by morphine receptors in the brain in preference to morphine and is able to displace morphine from these sites. This interaction is one which may be of benefit to the patient who has been tipped into respiratory failure by morphine, or the patient who has taken an overdose of an opiate drug.

Sometimes drugs interact at receptor sites in a more indirect fashion; in some instances the exact mechanism is not fully worked out although the interactions are clinically very important.

Alcohol with antihistamines, barbiturates and tranquillisers

The precise way in which alochol interacts with antihistamines, barbiturates and tranquillising drugs (such as diazepam and chlorpromazine) is not known. All of these agents are cerebral depressants and all are potentiated by the use of alcohol and may produce profound drowsiness. You should warn your patients receiving any of these agents to be careful in their use of alcohol. This is particularly important for those of them who drive or who work near moving machinery on a factory floor.

Interactions at the sites where drugs are metabolised

Many drugs are broken down or transformed in the liver or body tissues by special proteins called enzymes. There are two principal methods by which drug A may interfere with the breakdown of drug B:

1. Drug A can inhibit the enzymes necessary to transform drug B into inactive compounds, thus prolonging the activity of drug B
2. Drug A can increase the amount of drug B-metabolising enzymes and thus speed up removal of drug B activity from the body.

Both of these mechanisms produce interactions with potentially serious effects for patients.

Phenytoin and phenylbutazone

Phenylbutazone inhibits the activity of the enzymes that metabolise phenytoin in the liver. Epileptic patients who receive both drugs are therefore liable to become intoxicated with phenytoin and to display ataxia (staggering gait) and drowsiness unless the dose of phenytoin is reduced.

6-Mercaptopurine and allopurinol

Both of these may be given to patients with acute leukaemia. 6-mercaptopurine is an antimitotic agent (p. 206) and during treatment the leukaemic patient is liable to produce enormous quantities of uric acid as a result of the breakdown of purines from the leukaemia cells killed by this drug. There is a danger that the uric acid may block the kidneys producing the very serious complication of anuria. Consequently many doctors prescribe allopurinol which inhibits the enzyme xanthine oxidase which makes uric acid.

Unfortunately xanthine oxidase also inactivates 6-mercaptopurine and when allopurinol is given to these patients they are liable to develop very serious side effects unless the dose of 6-mercaptopurine is drastically reduced.

A large number of drugs have the capacity to increase drug-metabolising enzymes in the liver. The best known of these drugs are the barbiturates but some anticonvulsant drugs (p. 144) and the antituberculous agent rifampicin (p. 115) also share this property.

Barbiturates and oral anticoagulants

The following illustrative case serves as an example of this serious interaction.

Mr Barrett, a 34-year-old patient with mitral stenosis and atrial fibrillation, was admitted to hospital with sudden onset of weakness of the left arm and leg. He was not seriously ill but it was decided that he had developed a cerebral embolus as a result of a piece of clot in the left atrium being dislodged and entering the internal carotid artery. Accordingly anticoagulant treatment with warfarin was started. Because Mr Barrett had great difficulty sleeping at night owing to the noises emanating from a confused patient in the ward the house officer prescribed a barbiturate drug as a hypnotic.

Recovery was uneventful. Accordingly Mr Barrett was discharged, receiving oral anticoagulants. It was decided to continue this therapy for

6 months and he was given an appointment for the return clinic in 2 weeks' time. His anticoagulant control was very good while he was in the ward, although the dose needed to control him did seem a little on the high side.

On his return home Mr Barrett felt very well. He was eating well and sleeping soundly. There were no noises to disturb him at night as there had been in the ward and he did not need to take his sleeping pills. All went well until 8 days after his discharge when he suddenly developed a severe pain in his groin and upper thigh. The flesh there became tense, discoloured and very tender. Mr Barrett started to break out in a sweat and then rapidly lost consciousness. When he came round he was in the hospital once more receiving his third pint of blood. He had had a massive haemorrhage into the tissues of the thigh. Four pints of blood were required together with the administration of vitamin K to correct the very low level of prothrombin in the blood. Mr Barrett was in hospital for a further 2 weeks and was unwell with muscle pain and stiffness in the leg for 3 months after that. He was lucky however: he could have died.

What happened was this: the barbiturate hypnotic increased the amount of warfarin metabolising enzymes in the liver. This meant that Mr Barrett broke down his warfarin more rapidly than normal and so needed a higher dose to produce the therapeutic effect. On returning home he stopped barbiturates and the activity of warfarin-metabolising enzymes in the liver rapidly returned to normal. But he was still taking a relatively high dose of anticoagulant. The next few days witnessed accumulation of warfarin in the blood to dangerously high levels with the inevitable development of spontaneous haemorrhage.

Barbiturates must not be given to patients on anticoagulant therapy; nor should the hypnotics glutethimide and dichloralphenazone as they act in a fashion similar to barbiturates. Nitrazepam does not cause an increase in drug-metabolising liver enzymes and is therefore a safe hypnotic in this respect.

SUMMARY OF SOME IMPORTANT AND POTENTIALLY DANGEROUS INTERACTIONS

1. Aspirin and phenylbutazone increase the effect of warfarin, tolbutamide, chlorpropamide and methotroxate (by displacing these substances from plasma albumen)
2. Sulphonamides increase the hypoglycaemic effects of chlorpropamide and tolbutamide (by displacing these drugs from plasma albumen)

3. Barbiturates accelerate the metabolic inactivation of warfarin, phenylbutazone, phenytoin and griseofulvin, thus hindering the attainment of effective therapeutic plasma levels. This is potentially dangerous in the case of warfarin when barbiturate therapy is stopped
4. Monoamine oxidase inhibitors (p. 143) increase the effect of such drugs as amphetamines. They also increase the liability to develop toxic responses to the substance tyramine in cheese, meat extracts and red wine by inhibiting enzymes which normally inactivate these substances
5. Imipramine and amitriptyline antagonise the hypotensive action of adrenergic blocking drugs such as guanethidine and bethanidine
6. Drowsiness induced by barbiturates, antihistamines, chlorpromazine and related drugs, diazepam and antidepressants, is worsened by alcohol.

At the beginning of this chapter it was stated that modern drugs are really very safe. Having finished the chapter you would be forgiven for thinking that this was just not true! The truth which should now be apparent is that the drugs themselves are safe, it is the way in which they are used which is often not. It is not likely that you will remember all the adverse reactions mentioned in the chapter and it probably does not matter so long as you know how to obtain advice and assistance when the need arises. It is much more important that you realise that many of the reactions and interactions listed are 'avoidable'. Sensible use of drugs, selection of correct dosage and identification of the particular weaknesses of the patient (for instance, respiratory or hepatic failure) are actions which effectively prevent the majority of serious adverse drug effects.

Those of you who have already worked in the wards may think it strange that a chapter on adverse drug effects has so far failed to mention the typical example of the elderly patient admitted in a confused state who has been receiving nine different preparations, four of which are sedative drugs. This example has been kept to last as it is one of the most common and certainly one of the most important forms of drug toxicity. It must be obvious that academic considerations about potential drug: drug interactions are of no importance in this situation. Commonsense dictates that when several drugs are given to an elderly person problems are bound to develop solely as a result of the combined therapeutic effect of the different agents. More complicated explanations are simply not necessary. Sedative drugs are the usual culprits. Any sedative drug used alone in doses normal for a healthy adult is likely to lead to confusion in a proportion of elderly patients. Several sedative drugs used together will lead to more confusion. The answer to this problem is so obvious that it does not require stating. This is by no means a problem confined to prescribing outside hospital. Study the drug prescription charts of the average medical or surgical ward and you will find at least one octogenarian who is simultaneously receiving diazepam and chlorpromazine during the day and nitrazepam at night to aid sleep! The likelihood is that this patient will be discharged from hospital with a good supply of this toxic combination. The only hope then is that an enlightened general practitioner will stop the lot or that the patient's confusion will lead to the drugs being flushed down the toilet!

Far too many drugs are used both inside and outside hospital. Try to make a habit of deciding for yourself which drugs are really essential for each of the patients under your care and do not be afraid to question the need for any drug which seems unnecessary.

Appendix

DRUGS AND DOSAGES

A proprietary preparation of a drug is one which carries the brand name of a particular manufacturer. For example, Achromycin and Ambramycin are both proprietary names for the drug tetracycline, which is the non-proprietary or approved name. There is often more than one proprietary name for a drug and proprietary preparations are often, although not always, more expensive than approved preparations. To avoid confusion and minimise expense it is advisable to use approved names when speaking of drugs.

If you nurse in Great Britain you should make yourself familiar with the British National Formulary (B.N.F.) and with the Monthly Index of Medical Specialties (M.I.M.S.). Both of these should be available in all hospital wards and both are invaluable reference books for dosages and routes of administration of drugs and for the approved names of proprietary preparations.

Your legal position with regard to the handling and storage of Dangerous Drugs in hospitals in Great Britain is well summarised in the booklet *Law Notes for Nurses* by S. R. Speller, published by the Royal College of Nursing, Henrietta Place, Cavendish Square, London, W.1. Dangerous Drugs include such substances as morphine, opium and cocaine. They must be stored in a cupboard specially kept for the purpose, which must be locked. The key must be kept on the person of the ward sister (or in a theatre, the theatre sister) or on the person of an acting sister appointed by the sister in her absence. It is usually assumed that the person appointed as acting sister should be at least an enrolled nurse. Although not a statutory requirement, it is very important to keep an accurate note of all medicines given to patients in hospital. Use of the so-called Aberdeen system of prescribing from a drug kardex may help here and this system is being adopted in many hospitals. Prescriptions of Dangerous Drugs should state the amount of the drug given, the date and the time at which it was given and should be signed both by the nurse who gives the drug and the doctor who orders it. It is the practice in many hospitals to keep a special 'Dangerous Drugs book' for this purpose.

You should read the report of the Joint Sub-Committee on the Control of Dangerous Drugs and Poisons in Hospitals. This is published by Her Majesty's Stationery Office London. This booklet gives invaluable information of a commonsense nature on the nurse's statutory obligations in relation to Dangerous Drugs and poisons. Every nurse should read it.

Index